New Insights into Oral Health Science and Dentistry

New Insights into Oral Health Science and Dentistry

Editor: Victor Martinez

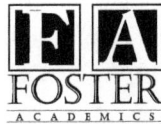

FA FOSTER
ACADEMICS

www.fosteracademics.com

www.fosteracademics.com

FA
FOSTER
ACADEMICS

Cataloging-in-Publication Data

New insights into oral health science and dentistry / edited by Victor Martinez.
    p. cm.
Includes bibliographical references and index.
ISBN 978-1-63242-612-3
1. Mouth--Care and hygiene. 2. Oral medicine. 3. Dental care.
4. Dental public health. 5. Mouth--Diseases. 6. Dentistry. I. Martinez, Victor.
RK60.7 .N49 2019
617.601--dc23

Foster Academics,
118-35 Queens Blvd., Suite 400,
Forest Hills, NY 11375, USA

ISBN 978-1-63242-612-3 (Hardback)

Contents

Permissions

List of Contributors

Index

Preface

I am honored to present to you this unique book which encompasses the most up-to-date data in the field. I was extremely pleased to get this opportunity of editing the work of experts from across the globe. I have also written papers in this field and researched the various aspects revolving around the progress of the discipline. I have tried to unify my knowledge along with that of stalwarts from every corner of the world, to produce a text which not only benefits the readers but also facilitates the growth of the field.

Oral health science is the practice of maintaining hygiene in one's mouth by keeping it clean and disease-free. Maintenance of oral hygiene on a regular basis is highly crucial for preventing bad breath and other dental diseases. Dentistry is a branch of medicine concerned with the study, diagnosis, prevention and treatment of diseases and conditions related to the oral cavity. Tooth decay, gingivitis and periodontitis are some of the common oral-hygiene related diseases. Regular brushing is required to prevent oral diseases. Apart from this, interdental cleaning plays an important role in cleaning the space between the teeth. Interdental brushes, floss and flossettes are some of the common tools used for the purpose of interdental cleaning. This book unfolds the innovative aspects of dentistry which will be crucial for the progress of this field in the future. The topics included herein on oral health science and dentistry are of utmost significance and bound to provide incredible insights to readers. For all readers who are interested in these areas, the case studies provided in this book will serve as an excellent guide to develop a comprehensive understanding.

Finally, I would like to thank all the contributing authors for their valuable time and contributions. This book would not have been possible without their efforts. I would also like to thank my friends and family for their constant support.

Editor

Ultrasonic Instrumentation

Ana Isabel García-Kass,
Juan Antonio García-Núñez and
Victoriano Serrano-Cuenca

1. Introduction

Although ultrasounds (US) were discovered in the 18th Century due to their use in animal kingdom, they were not manufactured until the 19th Century, when certain devices facilitating the reproduction of these non audible for human sounds were developed. They constitute rare frequencies with several properties. First of all they were developed for their use in navy and in medicine. In the 20th Century it was noticed that they could have uses in dentistry, so the first applications for calculus removal were initiated, taking advantage of their mechanical energy and cavitation effect. The different possibilities achieved by conventional US together with those of sonicators, of lower frequency but with similar effects, resulted in a fast development of these technologies.

Since Michigan longitudinal studies demonstrated that the open flap radicular instrumentation techniques were in a long term as effective as the closed ones, the latter were developed, so treatment of periodontitis suffered a change of paradigm. From that moment on, periodontal treatment involved less open flaps and more mechanical treatments, limiting surgeries to very concrete cases, in order to enable access to the deepest pockets and furcations. The result was a reduction in discomfort for patients and a better long term prognosis. Prevention gained more importance and supportive periodontal therapies were regularly done adjusting them to the individual necessities of each patient, depending on the type of periodontitis and the severity of the case. To reduce the number of surgeries, it was crucial to develop instruments able to reach deep pockets. Small curettes and microcurettes were developed, and later on special ultrasonic tips which allowed the instrumentation of pockets of difficult access for Gracey and Universal curettes. Even when effectuating periodontal surgery, clinicians preferred US rather than curettes for the narrow furcations´ instrumentation. The fewer fatigue of the professional and the efficacy of the results have favoured the great development of these instruments during the last years.

A new progress occurred in dentistry with the introduction of piezoelectric US. These US produced less discomfort in patients, and with the development of special tips imitating microcurettes, deep and narrow pockets instrumentation was possible without doing surgery. With the important development of implant rehabilitations during the last twenty years and the subsequent peri-implantitis, the necessity of new instruments has arisen, as traditional and teflon curettes are not suitable for this purpose. To solve this problem, tips of teflon and other materials have emerged to facilitate the elimination of deposits settled over the irregular implants' surface, with controversial results.

The use of US in endodontics was introduced later to clean and disinfect root canals. It is quite useful basically to make easier the access to the root canals in certain conditions, in endodontic retreatments and to clean before the sealing of the root canal. One of the latest US applications in dentistry is in surgery, as they avoid discomfort of rotary instruments while preserving the soft tissues. The cut precision allows their use in implants' surgery, ostectomies and especially in those techniques where tearing of soft tissues could be produced due to their proximity, i.e., sinus lift procedures. These techniques are in continuous progress; they are linked to piezo-electric US and to those new materials allowing their use in favourable conditions.

The aim of this chapter is to revise the physical principles of US, the materials used and the historical evolution, their basic uses in perio and endodontics, as well as their efficacy when comparing with other techniques and finally the possibilities in maxilar surgery. Other less frequent applications are also mentioned.

2. History and physics of ultrasounds

Before 1700 man was unaware of ultrasounds because their frequency is below human's audible frequency. In 1700, Spallanzani described their use by bats when flying and capturing their preys. Later on, it was demonstrated that other animal species had the same faculties, and in the 19th Century, with the discovery of Doppler effect about deformation of light waves in movement, it was observed that this property could also be applied to ultrasounds. In fact, they are sound waves that are not audible for men due to their high frequency (Figure 1).

At the end of the 19th Century, the Curie brothers [1] described the piezoelectric effect (from greek *piezein*, mechanic pressure) of several crystals, property used later for the fabrication of ultrasonic devices with new characteristics. At this time, in 1883, Galton develops a high frequency whistle to find out the human hearing limit, and from that moment on ultrasounds (US) for different applications are developed. Although the first ultrasonic apparatus date from 1950, the first commercial application for dentistry was in periodontics in 1957 with Cavitron®, developed by Dentsply for doing prophylaxis and calculus removal. Its name comes from the cavitation effect produced by ultrasounds when working with water. When a liquid flows through a region where pressure is lower than its steam pressure, the liquid boils and produces

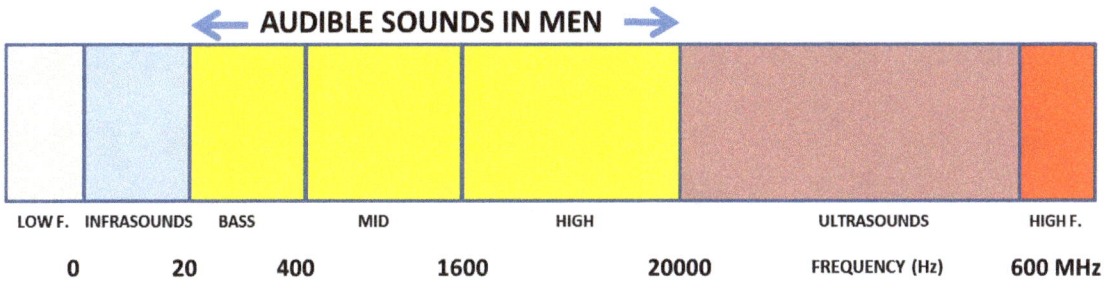

Figure 1. Human audition and ultrasound frequencies in Hz

vapour bubbles. The bubbles will be carried to a higher pressure area, where the steam returns immediately to the liquid phase, imploding the bubbles suddenly. Thus, a change from liquid to gaseous phase takes place, and again to liquid phase with water dissociation and formation of H^+ and OH^- (Figure 2).

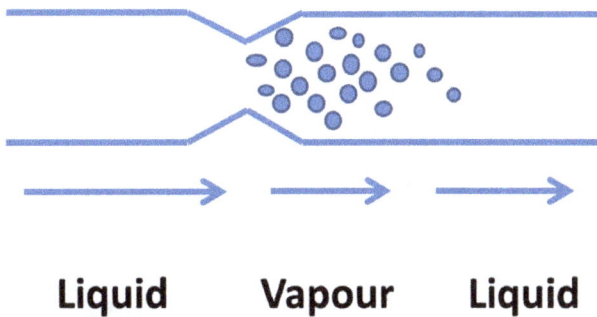

Figure 2. Representation of cavitation effect

Cavitation is defined as the formation of submicroscopic cavities or vacuums as a result of the vibration of a fluid due to the high frequency alternating movement of the tip of an instrument. When these vacuums implode, shock waves which spread through the medium are generated and produce energy (heat) release [2].

The basis of the ultrasonic action consists of an electric generator transmitting vibrations to the tip of the device with frequencies of 25,000 to 30,000 Hz, whose shock waves generate pressures and depressions which detach the calculus and break water molecules by the cavitation phenomenon. To the effect of cavitation it adds an acoustic streaming, with a great cleaning and bactericidal action, which potentiates the bactericidal effect of cavitation, effect that can increase adding an antiseptic product to the irrigation fluid.

There are two types of ultrasonic devices: the classical ones, laminated or magnetostrictive, with elliptical oscillation of the tip, and the piezoelectric ones, of quartz with lineal oscillation. Laminated US are based on the Joule magnetostriction phenomenon. According to this phenomenon, several ferromagnetic materials get deformed when they go through a magnetic field. The deformation degree depends on the material employed, the magnetization strength, the previous treatment of the material and the temperature. The metallic sheets are situated in the handle, i.e. in the handpiece where the insert is placed (Figure 3).

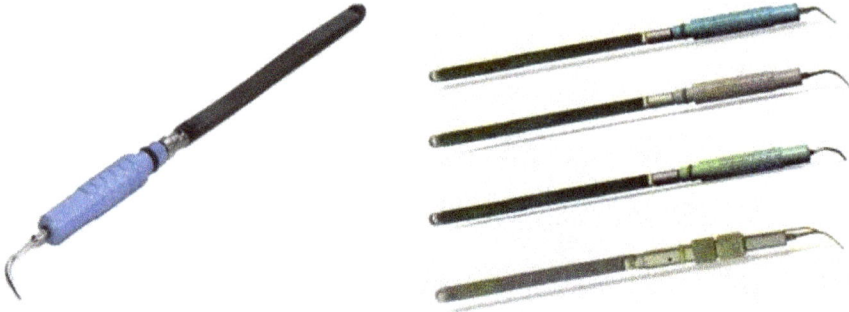

Figure 3. Laminated US device and several ultrasonic inserts for Cavitron

Piezoelectric US (Figure 4) are based on quartz clock principles. When applying an alternating current to the ceramic/quartz discs, changes in polarity produce expansion and contraction trasmitting the oscillation to the tip, applicator or insert. The sound thus generated, presents the same intensity, frequency and wavelength than the material employed in its fabrication (quartz, zinc blende, sodium borate...). Nowadays, the most used crystals are ceramic zirconate discs, which are less sensitive to temperature and blows.

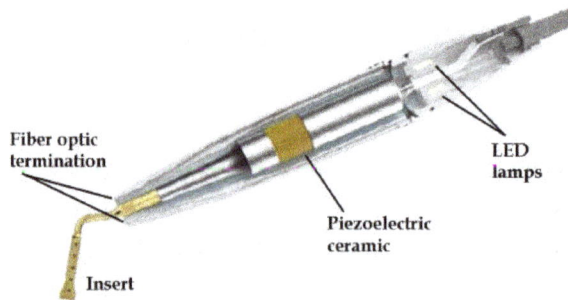

Figure 4. Piezoelectric US for surgery. Modified from Variosurg (NSK) catalogue

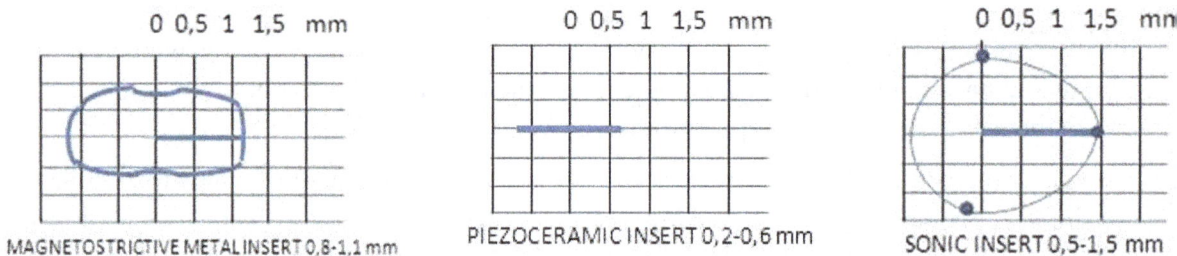

Figure 5. Oscillation of magnetostrictive US, piezoceramic US and sonicators

3. Biologic actions

US present several effects over the tissues which vary depending on the time, type of US and way of application. These effects are mechanical, thermal, biological, chemical, massage and placebo.

1. Mechanical effects. The most important, as vibration favours the removal of calculus, biofilm and of the cementum surface, damaged by bacterial toxins and sometimes contaminated by bacteria (Figure 6). Inside the root canals, US clean the pulpal detritus.

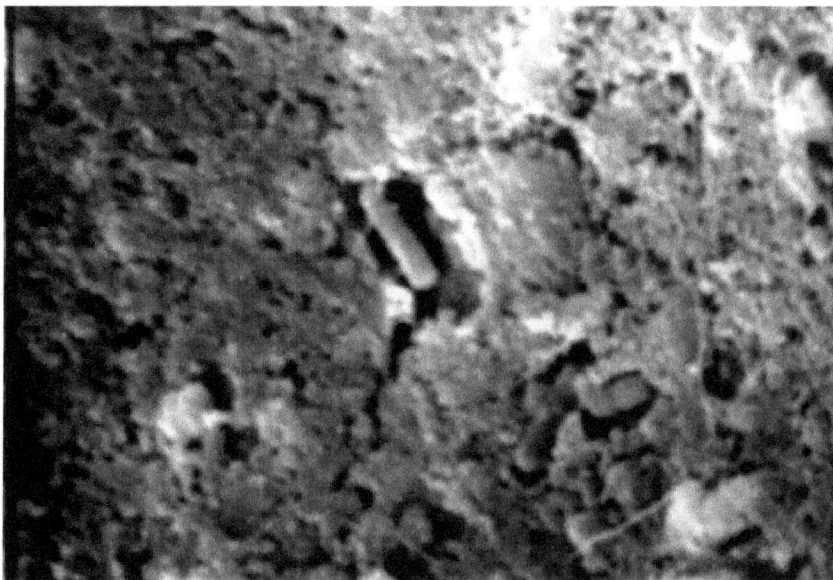

Figure 6. Bacterial presence inside cementum in periodontitis. Original magnification SEM x3000. Bacteria can be identified supragingivally, in the epithelial junction and in apical areas of cementum

2. Thermal effects. US are a way of energy and thus, during their application, heat is generated. This heat can be useful, as it favours the cleaning of the treated area and the elimination of detritus, blood debris, biofilm and calculus; but if it is excessive it could burn the tissues, especially gingiva and periostium. This is the reason why it is crucial to control the irrigation system, checking for possible obstructions of applicator/insert.

3. Biological effects. US produce an increase in permeability of the cellular membrane, known as phonophoresis, which facilitates the cellular function, and thus the recuperation of the inflamed soft tissues.

4. Chemical effects. Ultrasonic vibration favours the chemical processes in the area in which they are applied. Biological exchanges among the treated tissues improve; in addition, an increase of the blood supply takes place, helping to reduce inflammation and to facilitate the arrival of blood cells and anti-inflammatory mediators, favouring tissue normality. It

also produces oxidation and macromolecule depolymerization phenomena, due to the ions release.

5.   The massage and placebo effects, also associated to US, are of less interest in our field, but they should not be forgotten.

Due to the cavitation effect and the acoustic micro-streaming produced by oscillatory movements of ultrasonic inserts, US are used in humans in different ways for diagnosis and treatment. In the oral cavity they are mainly used for root instrumentation in periodontics, and less in endodontics, ostectomy, and sinus lift procedures. There are also other less frequent applications that we shall describe.

4. US in periodontics and implants

It is well known that periodontal disease is based on the presence of a mature biofilm with more than 700 bacterial species, being only a fraction of them related to periodontitis. The progression of the disease depends on the periodontopathogens, but also on the patient's immune system and its response to bacterial aggression. The elimination of bacteria, their toxins and calculus produced by saliva, is essential to keep under control the disease. Once local factors are removed, a strict hygiene is required, as well as a supportive periodontal treatment program, in order to eliminate calculus and subgingival biofilm, which is the main responsible of the bone and attachment loss and is formed shortly after its elimination.

Treatment was traditionally based on the mechanical elimination of plaque and calculus, which facilitate biofilm's survival, mainly using hand instruments and US, directly or by an open flap procedure. Longitudinal studies of the decades of 70's and 80's, showed that even most periodontally advanced cases, well treated and maintained, remained stable through the years [3], versus those patients who did not receive any treatment, who suffered a considerable tooth loss and worsening of periodontal parameters [4].

Since Michigan longitudinal studies [5-7] demonstrated that the open flap radicular instrumentation techniques were in a long term as effective as the closed ones [7], the latter were developed, so treatment of periodontitis suffered a change of paradigm. From that moment on, periodontal treatment involved less open flaps and more mechanical treatments, limiting surgeries to very concrete cases, in order to enable access to the most deep pockets and furcations [8]. The result was a reduction in discomfort for patients and a better long term prognosis. Prevention gained more importance and supportive periodontal therapies were regularly done adjusting them to the individual necessities of each patient, depending on the type of periodontitis and the severity of the case.

To reduce the number of surgeries, it was crucial to develop instruments able to reach deep pockets. Small curettes and microcurettes were developed, and later on special ultrasonic tips which allowed the instrumentation of pockets of difficult access for Gracey and Universal curettes.

The first device used in periodontal prophylaxis was Cavitron®, introduced in 1957 by Dentsply (USA). With the important development of implant rehabilitations during the last twenty years and the subsequent peri-implantitis, the necessity of new instruments has arisen, as traditional and teflon curettes are not suitable for this purpose. Ultrasonic instruments are very comfortable to use, they produce less fatigue in the operator than curettes and allow the combination of different tips and products in order to improve the treatment efficacy. Several authors [9] even demonstrate better results when instrumentation is done with US instead of curettes.

During the 80's, we demonstrated in several publications that prophylaxis done *in vitro* with US resulted at least equal or even more effective than with curettes [10, 11] (Figure 7).

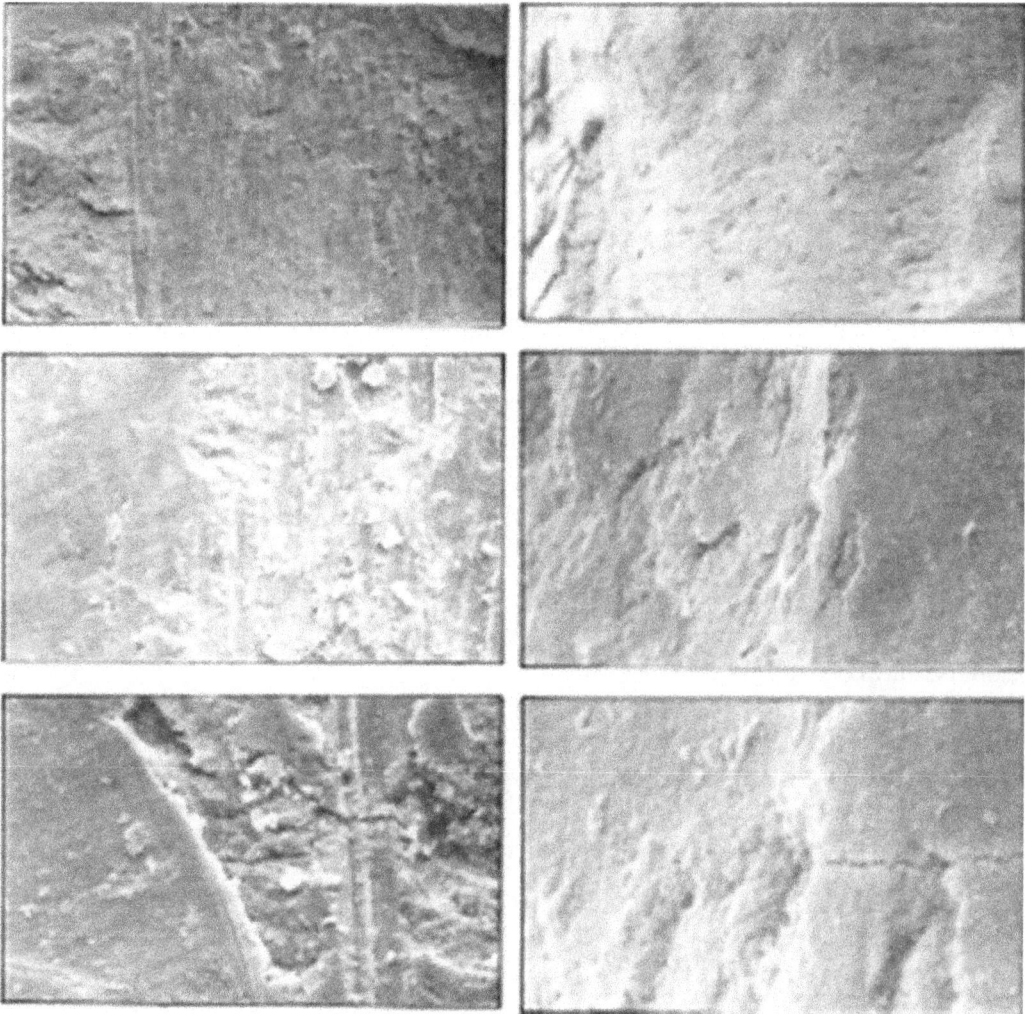

Figure 7. Cementum of the same tooth treated with curettes (left) and US (right). Original magnification SEM x352, x1136 and x3000

In Drisko's 1993 review, it is suggested that a thorough radicular debridement can be achieved without overinstrumentation, using certain sonic and ultrasonic scalers. The evaluation of residual plaque and calculus after hand and mechanical instrumentation with sonic and ultrasonic scalers, shows that sonic and US instruments obtain similar, and in some cases, better results than those obtained with manual instrumentation. When comparing modified ultrasonic inserts with unmodified ultrasonic inserts and manual scalers, it is observed that the modified ones generate smoother surfaces, better plaque and calculus removal, less damage and better access to the bottom of the pocket, which together with a less operating time lead to a lower fatigue [12].

Several years later, another review of the same author shows that US, through their cavitation effect, are able to eliminate toxins from the cementum surface without damaging it. This, together with the irrigation action, improves healing, as it is not necessary an excessive instrumentation of cementum to achieve satisfactory results. The additional benefits of the chemical irrigation during ultrasonic instrumentation are the weakly attached subgingival plaque removal and a better access to difficult areas such as narrow and deep pockets, root grooves and furcations. Thus, microultrasonic tips, of smaller diameter, allow the penetration 1 mm farther than manual instruments [13].

In a position paper of 2000, US and sonicators were compared, reaching similar results than hand instruments in terms of plaque, calculus and endotoxins removal. Ultrasonic scalers used at medium power produced less damage in root surfaces than manual instruments or sonicators. Furcations seemed to be more accesible when using sonic or ultrasonic scalers than when using manual instruments. It was still not clear if root roughness was more or less pronounced when using US or curettes, and if the roughness produced in radicular cement affected long term wound healing. Although the aim of root instrumentation is the highest as possible elimination of calculus and toxins, it is necessary to preserve cementum. According to the reviewed papers, toxins remain in the root surface, thus being easily removed with US. One of the main problems of the intervention with US and sonicators is the aerosols production, which involves the risk of transmitting infectious diseases, therefore it is essential the use of barriers against aerosols. Concerning the use of chemical agents there is no evidence of their additional clinical benefit [14].

To avoid the potential damage of the cementum surface done by sonic and US instruments and curettes, and looking after an effective treatment of the root surface, a sonic instrument covered by teflon was introduced in order to compare it with the standard instrumentation and with Per-io-Tor in extracted teeth. Per-io-Tor and the mentioned sonic instrument seemed to be adequate for soft deposits' elimination in the root surface, but not for calculus removal [15].

Another study compared *in vivo* the effect of two piezoelectric US, Vector scaler and Enac scaler, with a hand scaler. Instrumentation was completed until the obtaining of a hard surface. Roughness, amount of remaining calculus and loss of dental substance were examined by SEM. Vectorial US provided a smooth root surface with minimal dental substance loss [16].

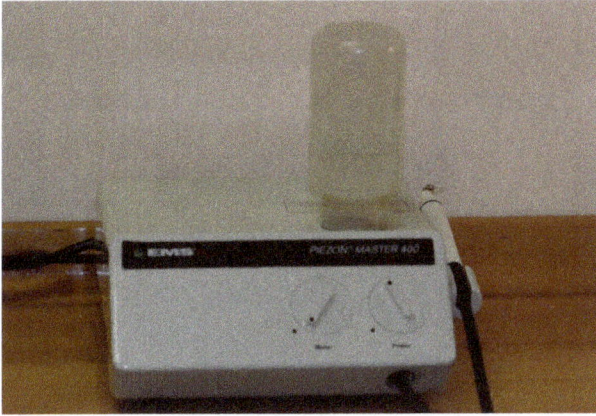

Figure 8. EMS piezoelectric US Piezon Master

The effects of US were described in 1969 by Clark [17]: they depend on the vibratory movement amplitude, the pressure applied, the instrument's tip sharpness, and the tip's application angle and time by surface unit. Their effects condition the way of use: they should be used at 40-50% of their power to avoid the metal fatigue and to favour the long-term duration of device and tip, they should be applied tangentially (parallel to the root surface) to avoid damage in the cementum surface (Figure 9), they should never be applied with the tip perpendicular to the cementum and the tip should be in a continuous movement (Figure 10) in order to avoid the production of holes in enamel and cementum. To avoid an excessive increase of temperature, the irrigation should be abundant (Figure 11), and to achieve an optimal efficacy the most suitable tip should be selected for each indication. It should be taken into account that it is different to work over a thick layer of supragingival calculus than over a thin subgingival layer, which is more adhered. This is the reason why large tips are used for superficial calculus, small tips for subgingival calculus, curette-like for scaling and thin and long for narrow and deep pockets (Figure 11).

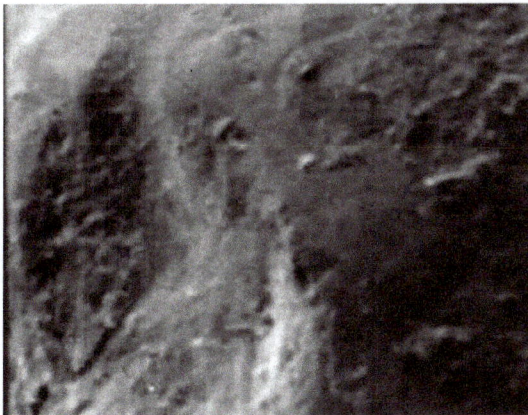

Figure 9. Hole in cementum due to a wrong ultrasonic instrumentation. Original magnification x600

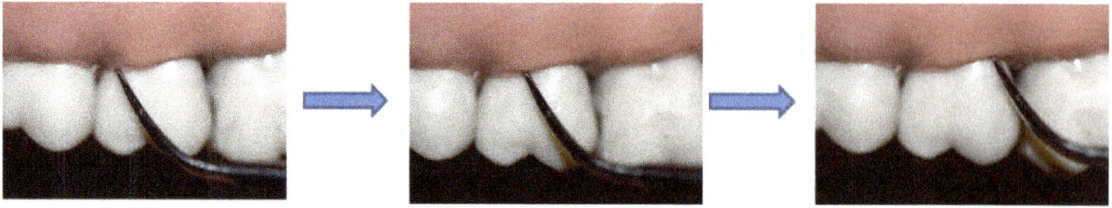

Figure 10. Insert application and displacement for calculus removal

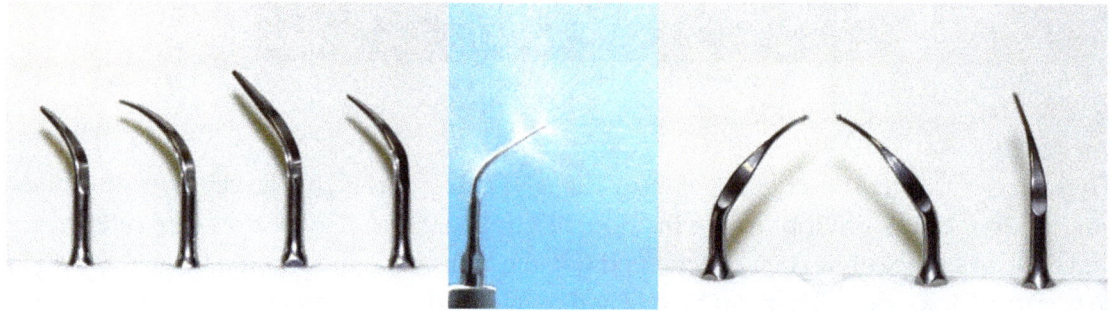

Figure 11. Supra (left) and thin subgingival (right) ultrasonic tips should always work with abundant irrigation

When US are used with complementary water tank and an antiseptic liquid, it is convenient to wash the whole circuit with demineralized water after its use, so the obstruction of tubes with the substances used is avoided. In case of using only water, it is recommended to fill in the deposit with low mineralized water, in order to facilitate the cleaning and prevent obstructions in tubes and inserts.

Due to their lineal oscillation over the dental surface, the actual rounded-tip piezoelectric US, reduce abrasion and obtain a uniform and smooth surface. With 32.000 oscillations per second, they are autoregulated and their cavitation effect and acoustic streaming reduce discomfort and have limited effects over gingival epithelium (Figure 12).

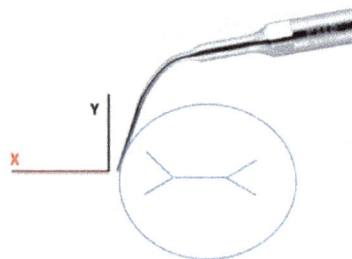

Figure 12. Vector decomposition of ultrasonic oscillation

Some of these US may incorporate two bottles, one for the bactericidal agent and the other for water for clearing or cleaning. They are also equipped with perio and endodontic tips.

Ultrasounds present few contraindications. They are not recommended in children except in very concrete cases. They should be avoided in the proximity of composite resins, as they could produce roughness or even detachment of the filling. They should not be used directly over ceramic partial fixed prosthesis or veneers, as ceramic could detach or break. In patients with certain types of pacemakers, interferences could be produced with inhibition and increase of the stimulation frequency. It is recommended the intermittent use of ultrasounds, avoiding the support of instruments over the generator as well as deprogramming the frequency modulation during the sessions. With a magnet, the pacemaker, which usually works at demand mode, converts into fixed-rate, not being sensitive to electromagnetic fields. In case of non sensible to electromagnetic interferences pacemakers, US could be used in the same way as in patients without pacemakers. Another option in these patients is the use of sonicators (Figure 13) because they use an air flow so they don't generate electromagnetic fields.

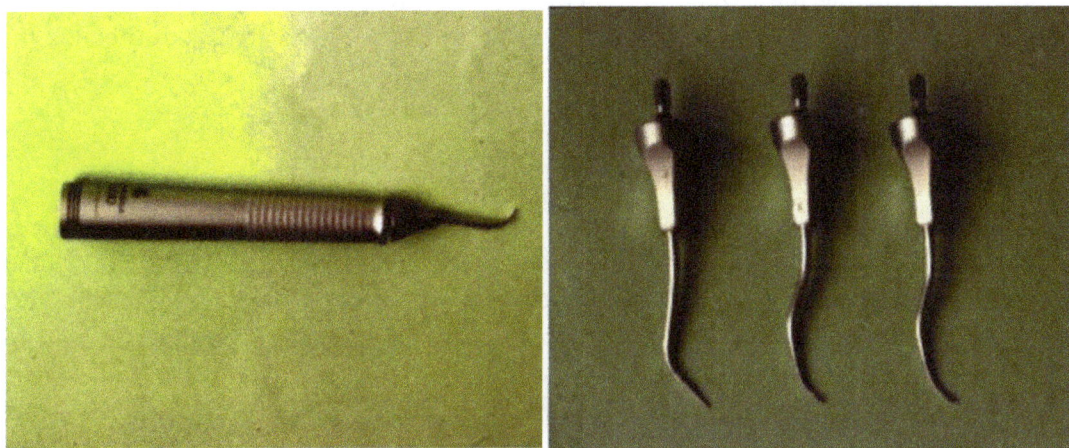

Figure 13. Sonicator and varied tips

These instruments present certain advantages and disadvantages in relation to ultrasounds. Their oscillation frequency is much lower, of 2,000 Hz, because the oscillation is produced by the air that arrives directly from the equipment and generates an orbital oscillation in the application tip. Their efficacy is similar to that of ultrasounds, but they can only use water instead of antiseptic liquids and the set of tips is much more reduced than the ultrasounds.

Ultrasounds are used as preventive and complementary to surgery treatment in implants. In this case the tip should not be metallic but of teflon, in order to avoid the damage of the implants´ surface (Figure 14).

Fox *et al.* compared plastic and metal curettes in titanium implants in an *in vitro* study. Plastic instruments produced an insignificant alteration of the implants´ surface after instrumentation, in contrast with metal instruments, which significantly altered this surface [18].

Something similar occurs when using Piezoelectric Ultrasonic Scalers with carbon, plastic and metallic tips on titanium implants. Remaining plaque and calculus index seemed to be similar with the three treatments. When using a laser profilometer and a laser scanning electron

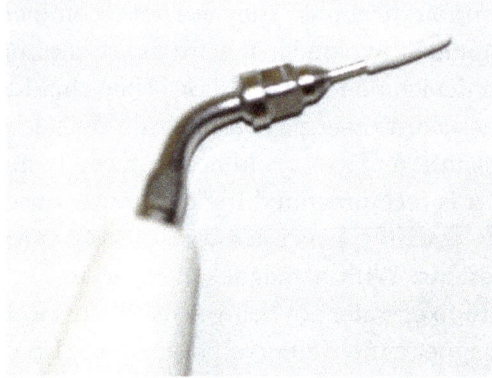

Figure 14. EMS Teflon insert for implants' instrumentation

microscope to evaluate the treated abutment surface characteristics, implants treated with carbon and plastic tips presented smoother surfaces than those treated with metallic tips, which were more damaged [19].

5. US in endodontics

US were incorporated into this field in 1957 when Richman used them for root canal cleaning and instrumentation [20]. In 1976, Martin improved endodontic treatment adding simultaneous irrigation, but its commercialization and use only were extended from 1980 by Martin *et al.* [21]. There are sonic apparatus in which special files are used, and several ultrasonic devices which work with standard files, with the usual colours and diameters (Figure 15).

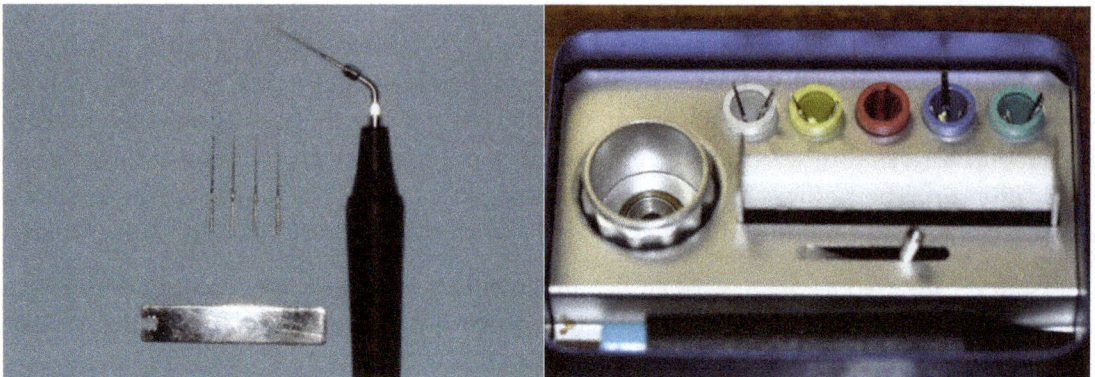

Figure 15. EMS ultrasonic handle and several endodontic K-files.

In endodontics US work by a transversal vibration, with a characteristic pattern of nodes and antinodes along the file's length (Figure 16) [22, 23], and may work in two different ways: with simultaneous ultrasonic instrumentation and irrigation (UI) or with passive ultrasonic irrigation (PUI), which works in an alternating way.

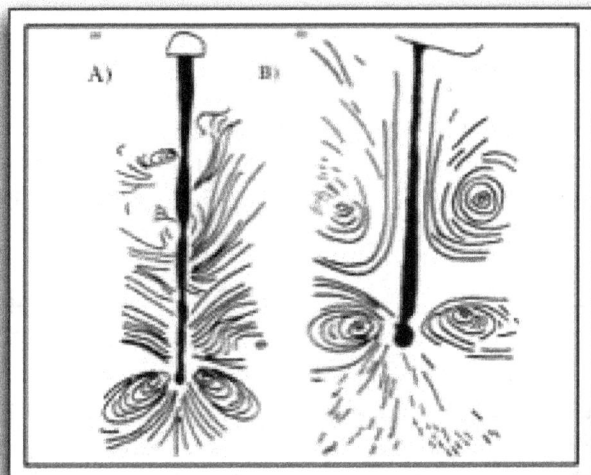

Figure 16. Diagrammatic representation of the current observed in ultrasonic (A) and sonic (B) activated files [24].

As for ultrasonic instrumentation UI, it is discussed if the root canals thus instrumented are significantly cleaner than those prepared with files in the usual way. Some authors support UI cleaning is better [25-29], while other studies affirm the cleaning is similar [30-36]. For Ruddle, these differences could be due to the limited space available in the root canal to let the ultrasonic vibration [37]. Also the lack of space could be responsible of the lesions produced during ultrasonic instrumentation, such as perforations and deficient root canal preparations [38]. This is the reason why this technique is only recommended after the complete root canal preparation [39], by what is known as PUI.

Passive ultrasonic irrigation was described by Weller [40] as a technique in which the effect of the ultrasonic tip reduces the risk of contact with the root canal surface, thus reducing the risk of perforation, while the cavitation and cleaning effects are preserved. As the root canal has already been prepared, the file moves freely and the irrigant penetrates easily in the apical area of the root canal system [41]. In this technique two ways of irrigation may be used: continuous or discontinuous, in which irrigation works intermittently after each ultrasonic cycle. Both of them allow control of irrigation, so they seem to be equally efficient [42].

Sonic instruments may also be used for root canal therapy with similar results. Jensen *et al.* compare the sonic and ultrasonic cleaning efficacy after manual instrumentation in molars with curved roots. Results are analysed with photomicrographs with a grid in order to quantify the debris and evaluate the root canal cleaning level in the three groups. Sonic and ultrasonic treated molars after manual instrumentation seemed to be cleaner than those only manually treated, while the level of cleaning among sonic and ultrasonically treated molars was similar [43].

Another recent *in vitro* study compares the ability of different ultrasound irrigation procedures to eliminate debris and to open the dentine tubules. Previously instrumented with mechanical rotatory technique single-rooted extracted teeth are treated with US. The amount of debris and the number of open dentinal tubules were established by SEM. In the apical third, ultrasonic activation of the irrigation with Irrisafe tips seemed to be the most effective method to eliminate debris and open dentinal tubules [44].

According to Martí-Bowen *et al.*, the use of US in periapical surgery with retrograde filling, it is feasible to reach difficult access root canals with sacrifice of few root tissue. Nowadays, good results are obtained in teeth with periapical pathology which previously were condemned to failure [45].

Van der Sluis *et al.* summarize the potential uses of US in endodontics with the following options: to improve the endodontic access (for example elimination of calcifications), irrigation of root canals, to remove broken posts and other obstructions inside the root canals, humectation with sealer of the root canal walls, guttapercha condensation of the obturations of root canals, mineral trioxide aggregate (MTA) application, endodontic surgery, and increase of the dentinal permeability in dental bleaching [46]; also to break fillings due to their shock effect, to remove old fillings and make easier the access to root canals, and in endodontic retreatments. There are available different applicators with the most adequate form for each use (Figures 17, 18).

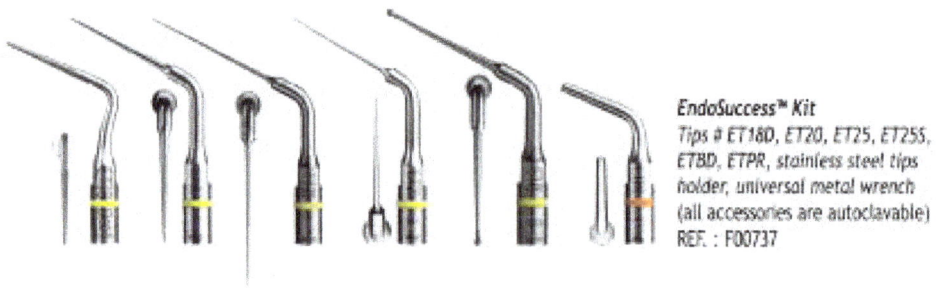

EndoSuccess™ Kit
Tips # ET18D, ET20, ET25, ET25S,
ETBD, ETPR, stainless steel tips
holder, universal metal wrench
(all accessories are autoclavable)
REF. : F00737

Figure 17. Satelec EndoSuccess Retreatment Kit. From left to right, tips for dentinal overhangs, calcificatons or filling materials elimination; for treatments in the coronal third; for treatments in the medium and apical thirds; for retreatment in coronal third and isthmus; for canal probing; and for loosening of posts and crowns. (Courtesy of Satelec, Merignac Cedex, France)

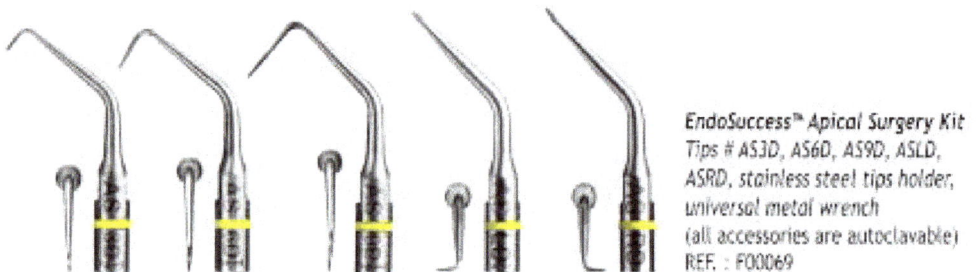

EndoSuccess™ Apical Surgery Kit
Tips # AS3D, AS6D, AS9D, ASLD,
ASRD, stainless steel tips holder,
universal metal wrench
(all accessories are autoclavable)
REF. : F00069

Figure 18. Satelec EndoSuccess Apical Surgery Kit. From left to right, universal apical surgery tip; second instrument; complicated cases (up to the coronal third), premolar left-orientated tip; premolar right orientated tip. (Courtesy of Satelec, Merignac Cedex, France)

6. US in surgery

Another application of US in dentistry is in oral and maxillofacial surgery to cut hard tissues. Experimental studies show that their application present better histological results than the rotary techniques. The precision of the cut with the different available inserts allows their use in our specialization in different fields such as general oral surgery, osseous grafts and implantology.

Although initially their use was reduced to sinus lift procedures, because they preserve the sinus membrane, their use has been extended to obtain bone grafts, osseous distraction and cortical split procedures, inferior dental nerve surgery, implant surgeries, extractions, etc. These biophotonic equipments allow changes in vibration's frequency from standard mode, with constant vibrations and frequency (used over soft tissues), to surgery mode (for hard tissues), where the modulation of amplitude and continuous vibration improves the efficacy over bone. Several applicators are designed for each osseous intervention (Figure 19).

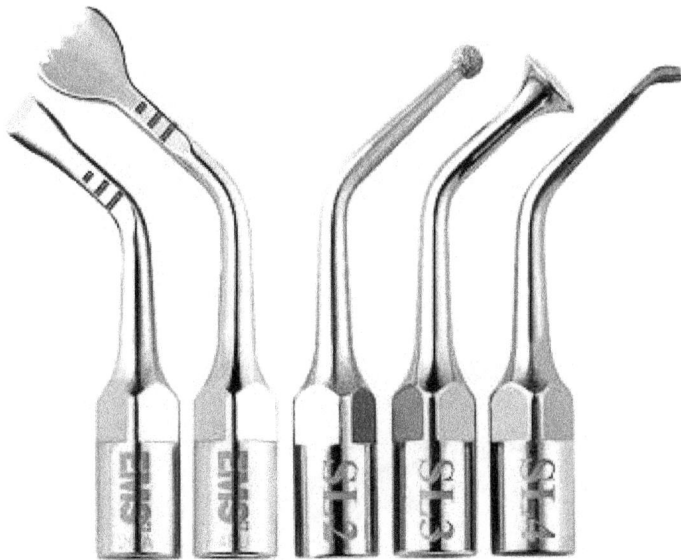

Figure 19. EMS Piezon Master Surgery US presents tips (from left to right) for vertical non-traumatic osseous incision, horizontal non-traumatic osseous incision, non-traumatic osteotomy, detachment of Schneider's membrane during sinus lift procedures and obtaining of bone fragments for bone augmentation.

The tips are different depending on the application: they present multiple lateral impact for surgery; curved, thin and scalpel-like for osteotomy; thin for non-traumatic extractions; cone-shaped diamond covered and calibrated for guiding during preparation; rounded or flat, diamond covered or scaler-shaped for sinus lift procedures. There are multiple surgical possibilities, as it is possible to do thin incisions for grafts, cysts elimination, sinus lift procedures with alveolar or lateral access, extractions, osteoplasties, osteotomies and other.

The advantages justifying their use are less bleeding and thus better visibility during the intervention, higher cut precision than with traditional instruments and less increase of temperature, less discomfort for patients as ultrasonic vibration is less noisy than drilling, and especially that the action over the soft tissues is minimal when they are accidentally applied over them, without tearing them up.

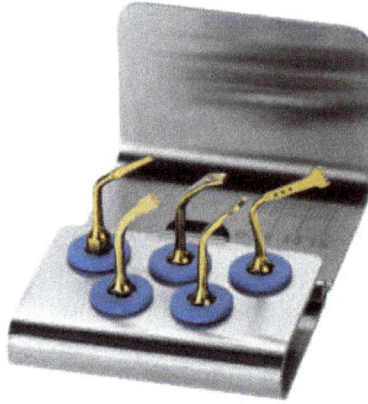

Basic Kit Piezosurgery

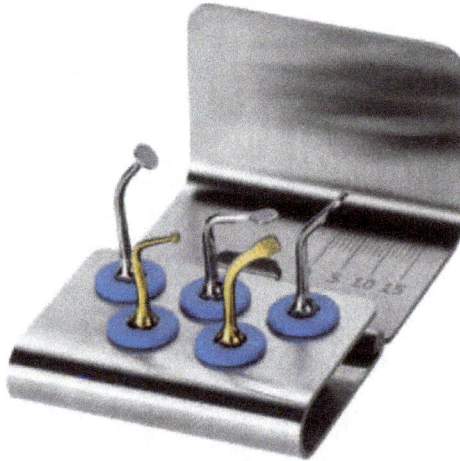

Figure 20. Mectron Piezosurgery's basic surgery and sinus lift procedure kits.

The action of the tip is effectuated by two mechanical effects: direct and indirect. In the direct mechanical effect, the tissues in contact with the tip are under a very high frequency. It is the effect of a hammer working only over the hard tissues. In the indirect one, positive and negative pressures are generated over the fluids; they are known as cavitation, and they displace the osseous tissue and potentiate the mechanical effects. This produces localized osseous destruction in a continuous or discontinuous way, being the surgeon who decides one or another possibility depending on the osseous density and the required refrigeration. This makes the cut selective without neither microscopic osseous nor soft tissue alterations. Refrigeration should be abundant with saline solution, in order to avoid heating and wash up the field to obtain a better vision.

Kits are usually available for each type of indication. The insert size and angulation allow the use depending on the necessities of the case. There are basic kits, kits for surgery, osseous distraction, implants, endodontic surgery, alveolar and lateral sinus lift procedures, osteoplasy and ostectomy, etc (Figure 20).

7. US trays

US trays deserve to be mentioned. Their utilization is essential in the dental office as intermediate step between the washing with soap and the sterilization of instrumental. They allow the elimination of organic debris that remain adhered in the instrument gaps facilitating the sterilization (Figure 21).

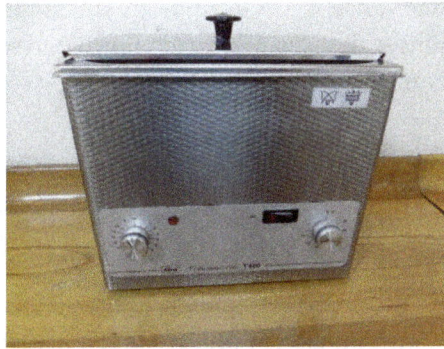

Figure 21. US tray.

Other applications of ultrasounds in Dentistry are removal of broken screws in implants, posts and crowns removal, etc. (Figure 22), but these applications are less frequent, they are not standardized and each professional acts according to his guidelines.

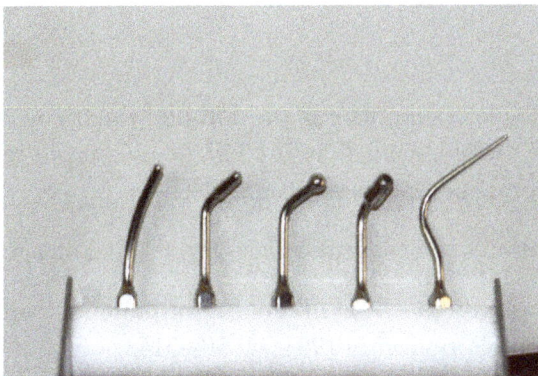

Figure 22. Set of diverse US tips

8. Conclusion

The evolution of US in dentistry during the last 65 years has been revised. The first laminated devices, only used for supragingival and slightly subgingival tartrectomies, have lead to sonicators and newer piezoelectric US with multiple inserts which allow the performance of tartrectomies reducing patient's discomfort and subgingival instrumentation. The variety of available tips lets us choose those which better adapt to our necessities and to the clinical situation, even in cases of periimplantitis. In endodontics, tips to facilitate the access, to clean the root canal and to carry out retreatments are available.

The industry offers the clinician optimal possibilities to achieve retrograde fillings more difficult or even impossible to carry out with other techniques. Among the latest applications, new possibilities emerge to effectuate certain surgical treatments, sinus lift procedures, implants placement, removal of fillings and crowns and other clinical situations.

Taking into account the great advance in US technology during the last years, it is reasonable to anticipate a great future for these devices. We are commited to regularly revisit the literature in order to know new opportunities provided by technology so the most suitable device is used in each clinical situation.

Author details

Ana Isabel García-Kass, Juan Antonio García-Núñez* and Victoriano Serrano-Cuenca

*Address all correspondence to: garcinu@odon.ucm.es

Department of Stomatology III, School of Dentistry, Complutense University of Madrid, Madrid, Spain

References

[1] Curie J, Curie P. Dévélopements par presión de l'électricité polaire dans les cristaux hémièdres à faces inclinées. In: Editeurs G-V, ed. Compte rendu hebdomadaire des séances de l'Académie des Sciences. Paris, 1880.

[2] American Association of endodontist Glossary, 6° Ed Chicago, 1998.

[3] Lindhe J, Nyman S. Long-term maintenance of patients treated for advanced periodontal disease. J Clin Periodontol 1984: 11: 504-514.

[4] Becker W, Berg L, Becker B. Untreated periodontal disease: a longitudinal study. J Periodontol 1979: 50: 234-244.

[5]   Ramfjord S, Knowles J, Nissle R, Shick R, Burgett F. Longitudinal study of periodontal therapy. J Periodontol 1973: 44: 66-77.

[6]   Knowles J, Burgett F, Nissle R, Shick R, Morrison E, Ramfjord S. Results of periodontal treatment related to pocket depth and attachment level. Eight years. J Periodontol 1979: 50:225-33.

[7]   Ramfjord S, Caffesse R, Morrison E, et al. 4 modalities of periodontal treatment compared over 5 years. J Clin Periodontol 1987: 14: 445-452.

[8]   Rateitschak-Pluss E, Schwarz J, Guggenheim R, Duggelin M, Rateitschak K. Non-surgical periodontal treatment: where are the limits? An SEM study. J Clin Periodontol 1992: 19: 240-244.

[9]   Matia J, Bissada N, Maybury J, Ricchetti P. Efficiency of scaling of the molar furcation area with and without surgical access. Int J Periodontics Restorative Dent 1986: 6: 24-35.

[10] Bascones-Martínez A, García-Núñez J, Herrera I, et al. MEB en superficies dentarias tratadas con diferentes aparatos de limpieza. Prof Dental 1983: 11: 5-12.

[11] García-Núñez J, Ramos-Navarro J, Cerero-Lapiedra R, Esparza-Gómez G. Resultado de las técnicas de profilaxis a la luz de la MEB. Av Odontoestomatol 1986: 7: 83-86.

[12] Drisko C. Scaling and root planing without overinstrumentation: hand versus power-driven scalers. Curr Opin Periodontol 1993: 78-88.

[13] Drisko C. Root instrumentation. Power-driven versus manual scalers, which one? Dent Clin North Am 1998: 42: 229-244.

[14] Drisko C, Cochran D, Blieden T, et al. Position paper: sonic and ultrasonic scalers in periodontics. Research, Science and Therapy Committee of the American Academy of Periodontology. J Periodontol 2000: 71: 1792-1801.

[15] Kocher T, Langenbeck M, Rühling A, Plagmann H. Subgingival polishing with a teflon-coated sonic scaler insert in comparison to conventional instruments as assessed on extracted teeth. (I) Residual deposits. J Clin Periodontol 2000: 27: 243-249.

[16] Kawashima H, Sato S, Kishida M, Ito K. A comparison of root surface instrumentation using two piezoelectric ultrasonic scalers and a hand scaler in vivo. J Periodontal Res 2007: 42: 90-95.

[17] Clark S. The ultrasonic dental unit: a guide for the clinical application of ultrasonics in dentistry and in dental hygiene. J Periodontol 1969: 40: 621-629.

[18] Fox S, Moriarty J, Kusy R. The effects of scaling a titanium implant surface with metal and plastic instruments: an in vitro study. J Periodontol 1990: 61: 485-490.

[19] Kawashima H, Sato S, Kishida M, Yagi H, Matsumoto K, Ito K. Treatment of titanium dental implants with three piezoelectric ultrasonic scalers: an in vivo study. J Periodontol 2007: 78: 1689-1694.

[20] Richman R. The use of ultrasonics in root canal therapy and root resection. Med Dent J 1957: 12: 12-18.

[21] Martin H, Cunningham W, Norris J, Cotton W. Ultrasonic versus hand filing of dentin: a quantitative study. Oral Surg Oral Med Oral Pathol 1980: 49: 79-81.

[22] Walmsley A. Ultrasound and root canal treatment: the need for scientific evaluation. Int Endod J 1987: 20: 105-111.

[23] Walmsley A, Williams A. Effects of constraint on the oscillatory pattern of endosonic files. J Endod 1989: 15: 189-194.

[24] Lumley P, Walmsley A, Laird W. Streaming patterns produced around endosonic files. Int Endod J 1991: 24: 290-297.

[25] Cunningham W, Martin H. A scanning electron microscope evaluation of root canal debridement with the endosonic ultrasonic synergistic system. Oral Surg 1982: 53: 527-531.

[26] Cunningham W, Martin H. Endosonics-the ultrasonic synergistic system of endodontics. Endod Dent Traumatol 1985: 1: 201-206.

[27] Stamos D, Sadeghi E, Haasch G, Gerstein H. An in vitro comparison study to quantitate the debridement ability of hand, sonic, and ultrasonic instrumentation. J Endod 1987: 13: 434-440.

[28] Lev R, Reader A, Beck M, Meyers W. An in vitro comparison of the step-back technique versus a step-back/ultrasonic technique for 1 and 3 minutes. J Endod 1987: 13: 523-530.

[29] Archer R, Reader A, Nist R, Beck M, Meyers W. An in vivo evaluation of the efficacy of ultrasound after step-back preparation in mandibular molars. J Endod 1992: 18: 549-552.

[30] Reynolds W, Madison S, Walton R, Krell K, Rittman B. An in vitro histological comparison of the step-back, sonic, and ultrasonic instrumentation techniques in small, curved root canals. J Endod 1987: 13: 307-314.

[31] Goldman M, White R, Moser C, Tanca J. A comparison of three methods of cleaning and shaping the root canal in vitro. J Endod 1988: 14: 7-12.

[32] Baker M, Ashrafi S, Van Cura J, Remeikis N. Ultrasonic compared with hand instrumentation: a scanning electron microscope study. J Endod 1988: 14: 435-440.

[33] Pugh R, Goerig A, Glaser C, Luciano W. A comparison of four endodontic vibratory systems. Gen Dent 1989: 37: 296-301.

[34] Walker T, del Río C. Histological evaluation of ultrasonic and sonic instrumentation of curved root canals. J Endod 1989: 15: 49-59.

[35] Ahmad M, Pitt Ford T, Crum L. Ultrasonic debridement of root canals: acoustic streaming and its possible role. J Endod 1987: 13: 490-499.

[36] Goodman A, Reader A, Beck M, Melfi R, Meyers W. An in vitro comparison of the efficacy of the step-back technique versus a step-back/ultrasonic technique in human mandibular molars. J Endod 1985: 11: 249-256.

[37] Ruddle C. Endodontic disinfection: tsunami irrigation. Endo Prac 2008: 2008: 7-16.

[38] Lumley P, Walmsley A, Walton R, Rippin J. Effect of precurving endosonic files on the amount of debris and smear layer remaining in curved root canals. J Endod 1992: 18: 616-619.

[39] Zehnder M. Root canal irrigants. J Endod 2006: 32: 389-398.

[40] Weller R, Brady J, Bernier W. Efficacy of ultrasonic cleaning. J Endod 1980: 6: 740-743.

[41] Krell K, Johnson R, Madison S. Irrigation patterns during ultrasonic canal instrumentation. Part I. K-type files. J Endod 1988: 14: 65-68.

[42] van der Sluis L, Gambarini G, Wu M, Wesselink P. The influence of volume, type of irrigant and flushing method on removing artificially placed dentine debris from the apical root canal during passive ultrasonic irrigation. Int Endod J 2006: 39: 472-476.

[43] Jensen S, Walker T, Hutter J, Nicoll B. Comparison of the cleaning efficacy of passive sonic activation and passive ultrasonic activation after hand instrumentation in molar root canals J Endod 1999: 25: 735-738.

[44] Mozo S, Llena C, Chieffi N, Forner L, Ferrari M. Effectiveness of passive ultrasonic irrigation in improving elimination of smear layer and opening dentinal tubules. J Clin Exp Dent 2014: 6: 47-52.

[45] Martí-Bowen E, Peñarrocha-Diago M, García-Mira B. Periapical surgery using the ultrasound technique and silver amalgam retrograde filling. A study of 71 teeth with 100 canals. Med Oral Patol Oral Cir Bucal 2005: 10: 67-73.

[46] van der Sluis L, Cristescu R. Ultraschall in der Endodontie. Die Quintessenz 2009: 60: 1281-1292.

Periodontal Changes and Oral Health

Petra Surlin, Anne Marie Rauten,
Mihai Raul Popescu, Constantin Daguci and
Maria Bogdan

1. Introduction

Periodontal disease is represented by inflammatory processes that affect the tooth's support / anchoring system and lead to tooth loss and negative effects on the oral health. Tooth loss and decreasing number of contacts between antagonist teeth was placed in relation to the educational level, marital status and incomes. Changes in periodontal status have been associated with oral factors and different systemic diseases.

2. Oral factors and periodontal changes

2.1. Caries, edentation and occlusal trauma

Maxillary represents a morphofunctional very complex entity, consisting of various components whose smooth work ensures performance of specific key like mastication, phonation, physiognomy and self-preservation, contributing in the same time, cooperation with other organs and tissues, to swallowing and respiration.

All physiological interrelationships of the components of the ensemble: the jaws including teeth with periodontal tissues, buccal mucosa, tongue, salivary glands, temporomandibular joint, neuromuscular complex and the veins that irrigate the functional territory providing nutrition, are directed by the central nervous system [1,2]. This dependence is due to the permanently received information by cortex from the entire reception network of maxillary. It satisfies the balance and health of each organ this way, in which the occlusion coordinates integrates.

It is acknowledged that any pain occurred in the maxillary area generated by a traumatogenic occlusion occurs not only locally, but also away from the mouth. Any alteration occurred in one of the components of the maxillary (under the action of certain triggers cumulated with the favoring ones), happens on a common ground: occlusion. On the other hand, disorganisation at the dental arches level, with a disruption of movement, can affect one of the elements of the same assembly, occurring dysfunctional disorders.

As teeth are dependent on their supporting tissues which keep them in the pockets of the maxillary bones, the periodontal complex depends on the activity of dental arches, normal occlusal function leading to a morphofunctional mechanical stimulation that manages the responsible biological mechanisms for the proper integrity of the periodontium [3].

The analysis of functional occlusion should be used as the basis for all conservative dental treatment, periodontal, prosthetic and orthodontic surgery.

Due to the functional differentiation structure of periodontal tissues and topographical situation of the two components (shell and supportive) defenses and resistance against aggressive risk factors direct or indirect is special, being conditioned by their character. On periodontal coating will act primarily micro-irritation local agents and at the periodontal support component factors of functional order, resulting dysfunction appearance. Risk factors that contribute to the disturbance or alteration action of periodontal can be classified into three big categories:

i.   General favorable factors with dysmetabolic character that alters nutrition of the body, including the marginal periodontium.

ii.   Local disturbing or precipitating factors that can be very divers, responsible for local trophicity change of periodontium.

iii.   Aggravating regional factors that alter regional trophicity due to the presence of mandibular dysfunction caused by premature occlusal contacts and interference.

Studies performed on occlusal function and dysfunction shows that traumatic dental pain can be caused by traumatic injury to periodontal, cracks or fractures of teeth vital and a change of direction forces acting on periodontal dental units [1].

The occlusion was defined as the ratio of static contact between the two arches, regardless of the position occupied by the jaw to the cranium, unlike the interdental articulation, which requires dynamic contact of the dental arch.

Dynamic occlusal reports are made by the two arches during the performance of the stomatognathic system and during parafunctions. Occlusion is considered one of the three determinants of mandibular dynamics. In the same time, occlusion shows a anterior determinant (the front arches) and a posterior determinant (the arch side), between which there is a balance and interaction summarized in the context of mutual protection. Under this concept between the two determinants of occlusion there is a mutual protection, acting on static and dynamic phases of occlusion [4].

Dental occlusion is meant to stabilize the mandible position to the skull, participating in the development of systemic functions. Occlusal disorders occur as a result of dental anomalies of number, volume, position, dental crown injuries, dental migrations, edentulous, change of occlusion parameters, and secondary musculoskeletal joint dysfunction. Clinically it manifests as premature contacts (characterized by occlusion static phases), occlusal interference (in mandibular dynamic with dental contact), localized abrasion (at a tooth or dental group that takes over occlusal) or generalized to the whole arch.

Occlusal contacts can occur in the static and dynamic positions the jaw. Any occlusal contact that prevents uniform coaptation of support areas and occlusal contact points is called premature occlusal contact. Occlusal contact occurs early in the static occlusion (at the end of the terminal occlusion trajectory), or in the dynamic occlusion when the path of the jaw movement interferes with the dental contact.

Premature contact is always traumatizing for stomatognathic system elements. Traumatogenic capacity of a contact point depends on several factors such as the point of contact location, the size of the contact point, the state of the contact surfaces [5].

This way, if the point of contact is on a bigger surface, the friction force increases with it, and its pathogen potential. A reduced in size contact point, but between two rough surfaces can be as traumatic or even more than one big point on a polished surface, due to the high friction coefficient. Contacts may be multiple and symmetrical, while maintaining the mandible in a position close to or almost identical to the centric relation or intercuspation position without deviations above it, the rear or side. This rarely happens because the presence of small occlusal contacts creates what is called an occlusal instability. Clinical evaluation of static and dynamic occlusion cannot be made without registration cranio-mandibular relations. Within the tendency to establish maximum intercuspation contact (in patients with long-centric) and centric occlusion (in patients with point-centric), jaw moves from rest position, rising to the jaw with the action of high muscles [4].

Dynamic occlusion analysis is performed through a test movement printed to the jaw, and also during mastication, phonation and deglutition movements. The analysis of the test movements (retrusion, protrusion, left and right laterality) often reveals the presence of occlusion blockages or of some traumatic sliding slopes. The retrusion movement performed between maximum intercuspation and centric relation can be blocked by some premature contacts, thus preventing the mandible excursion to centric relation during deglutition. The protrusion can register early contacts in the lateral area which would prevent the previous guidance of the occlusion on the retro incisive slope. The deeper is the occlusion, the larger is the trajectory of the protrusion. The premature contact points of the previous area in the protrusion movement prevent balanced contact of the whole frontal group in the guide movement, creating an overload of the teeth which keep the contact [6].

The test movements with left and right side orientation can reveal an inequality of the trajectories due to movement blocking through occlusal obstacles or due to their different orientation depending on the inclined planes which produce them. In the laterality movement there is recorded the most intense traumatogenic activity at the level of the interferences that may occur on the inactive or swing area, by turning the mandibular into lower grade leverage, therefore, more traumatic. In many cases, laterality or protrusion movement also causes a slight mobilization of the teeth which are in premature contact [4].

Occlusal force action on periodontal unit depends on the intensity, duration, direction of force, and the effects are also influenced by the state of tissue over which the force acts. The periodontal occlusal trauma is the degenerative injury that occurs when the occlusal forces exceed the adaptive capacity of the supporting tissue. Given that the dento-dental gearing is a cusp – fossa kind, the efforts leading is made in the long axis of the teeth. In normal circumstances, this condition is achieved by the way in which the teeth are implanted in the dental alveoli since their arcade eruption and through the manner in which are realized the dento-dental contacts in centric relation and maximum intercuspation, moments in which the masticatory pressures are maximum. In the teeth and periodontal tissue normal function, a particular importance has the correct position of dental organs, this being possible due to the presence of the balance between the multiple factors that are interrelated (presence of dental arcade integrity, the nature of the existing relations between adjacent teeth through contact areas and their character, dental morphology and cusps inclination, physiological mesial migration of teeth, physiological abrasion of teeth and their axial tilt, biological resistance of the healthy periodontium, lips, cheeks and tongue tone.

In the moment of integrity loss of dental arches, there occur multiple changes not only in the expense of odonto-periodontal units, but also for other components of the stomatognathic system, which demonstrates once again the present physiological interrelations between constituents of the complex.

Closely related to biomechanical homeostasis specific of the periodontium, the whole structural complex of the dento-maxillary system is conditioned by a series of morphological and functional elements that fit in the principle of inclined planes, among which the most important ones would be:

- Maximum and proximal vestibule-oral convexities of teeth ensure self-defense and self-stimulation of marginal periodontium through its protection against micro traumas that occur during mastication.

- The specific morphology of the frontal inferior teeth, vestibule-oral flattened in the third incisal and mesial-distal cervical narrowed to align them in a circle, defends the periodontium from pressures coming from the vestibule to the oral.

- Teeth roots' number and conical shape avoid the uneven application of the cementum-alveolar walls.

- Oral tilt of lower molars and vestibular tilt of the upper ones direct the masticatory pressures in the axial direction of these teeth while concentrating inwards massive facial.

When masticatory pressures are routed and transmitted in the long axis of the teeth, the ligaments that form the periodontal membrane are not crushed, but they act almost entirely, and are subject to forces with functional direction that determine their uniform extent, in functional limits with trophic effect on alveolar bone. After force's cessation, ligaments return to their spiral resting shape [7]. Taking into account that masticatory pressures are not permanent, periodontal ligaments are submitted to a real functional gymnastics, functional tasks interspersed with periods of rest, which stimulates periodontium, periodontal membrane and alveolar bone, and keeps it in normal parameters.

Local causes of traumatic occlusion with its negative consequences on the dento-maxillary are varied:

• Untreated caries, besides pulpal and periapical complications, they may also lead to occlusal disharmony and dysfunction by horizontal migration of proximal caries teeth or of their neighbors disturbing occlusal curves, vertical migration of antagonist teeth, of one tooth with occlusal caries or which considerably reduced the height of its crown, tipping of neighboring or antagonist caries teeth.

Through the loss of interdental contact point due to proximal caries, the fibrous foods can directly damage the marginal periodontium, which leads to periodontal damage and possible installation of a secondary occlusal trauma.

• The edentation without prosthesis acts by cancelling the dental arches continuity, due to loss of contact points, interrupting the continuity of the over alveoli ligaments system that normally form a connecting strap between teeth.

Also, the horizontal migration of teeth which border the edentulous breaches makes possible the spaces appearance between teeth and traumatic food impact of interdental gums papillae.

• Dental iatrogenic is often represented by inadequate fillings, inappropriate prosthetic marginal axial or transversal or which does not restore correctly proximal contact surfaces or natural convexities vestibule-oral and /or determine at the level of soft tissue rejection reactions, caused by prosthetic material.

The erroneous occlusal articular balancing compromised by grinding the occlusal stops and slopes guide altering vertical occlusal dimension and interdental space also produce occlusal dysfunction.

• Alteration of the morphology of dental crowns by pathological abrasion produces a broadening of the occlusal plane, constituting a cause of overload of odonto-periodontal units by masticatory forces.

• Primary malposition of some permanent teeth which erupt vicious in the three spatial planes. In this category, there are included anomalies of position: infra, over, predental, retrodental, vestibular or oral of some teeth, different combinations of malposition: mesio-vestibular position and distovestibular position.

• Isolated dental anomalies of form and volume can be generating occlusal interference by inconsistencies that appear in reports to other normally developed teeth. It produces a change in the position of teeth, bone implant base change, changing cuspid plans finally affecting occlusion reports.

- Occlusal vicious habits and tics are multiple and a source of risk factors for a dysfunctional maxillary. The most common harmful habits are: onychophagy (nail biting), biting objects (pipe, rubber, glasses frames), the practice of keeping and tighten between teeth, needle, nails, pencil, while working.

- Dentoalveolar fractures or maxillary bones may lead to dysfunctional occlusal interference. When the traumatic accident caused significant displacement of bone fragments of jaw, they rarely can be reduced in such a manner that there will be no significant occlusal changes after consolidation.

- Multiple parafunctions are the most common sources of occlusal dysfunction, bruxism holding priority. It is conditioned by the existence of occlusal disharmonies caused by premature dental contacts and occlusal interferences with an important role for multi-causal dysfunctional factors of the maxillary.

With a change of direction of force, normal pressure of normal muscle contractions become traumatic for periodontal membrane crushed between the tooth and alveolar wall it has no irrigation and normal metabolism anymore, and on the other hand, not all ligaments take functional tasks. Besides periodontal membrane suffering appears a harmful effect on alveolus: pressure causes bone lysis. Bone lysis always occurs in the way the force that causes pressure on the bone acts, which results in a stronger inclination of the tooth, like this appears traumatic periodontal conditions. By tilting the teeth it can escape the occlusal pressures making even dental contact to disappear; periodontal pain does not disappear with the disappearance of dental tooth contact as lack of stimuli periodontium undergoes hyaline degeneration of hypofunction [8]. Following these considerations to set the concept of primary occlusal trauma which means the harmful effect of occlusal forces on initial healthy periodontal when the direction, intensity or duration of occlusal force are beyond functional parameters: direction outside the long axis of the tooth, too long time, too much intensity. In this context, it should be emphasized that most studies are in agreement that the primary occlusal trauma (in the absence of superimposed etiologic factors, inflammatory, degenerative-dystrophic) does not causes periodontal disease but isolated periodontal lesions. Experience has shown that when the periodontium is weakened, initial periodontal suffering having other causes than occlusal, occlusal requests, even with optimal direction, the long axis of the teeth, even if they are intermittent, or even if the intensity normal, all lead to a periodontal trauma [9,10,11]. In this case, it is a secondary occlusal trauma in which the occlusal forces act on a previously weakened tooth periodontium. Obviously for already weaken teeth periodontium faulty forces within that direction, intensity or duration, have bad effects. Great difficulty occurs when, after periodontal is affected by an occlusal trauma, inflammatory component is superimposed, because at the moment it is hard to tell whether it is a primary or secondary occlusal trauma.

We can describe the three stages of occlusal trauma: stage of aggression, stage of repair and periodontal adaptation stage. During the stage of aggression collagen and osteogenic activity is inhibited, so that when the injury is not too strong to stimulate repair possibilities. If the trauma is not excessive, overcoming repair potential has serious periodontal consequences. If trauma is not excessive, it can reach the third stage, the periodontal adaptation. [12].

Disorders at the level of occlusive parameters characterized by shortening and cutting of occlusal areas, their artificial or mixed incorrectly realization, discontinuities, incorrect reconstructions of retroincisal slope, changes in the integrity and shape of support and guidance cusps, altered occlusion curves, uneven occlusal plane, are important factors of occlusal dysfunction, resulting in changes in jaw dynamic patterns, with muscle and joint response, taking into account the role of the dental determinant in achieving mandibular dynamics.

It is worth noting that the teeth in occlusal trauma, especially those with pathological abrasion, fractures may occur in low varnish areas, which can go up to an aspect of,, shelling " of dental crown [4].

True cuneiform lesions (mylolysis) are missing carious dentin being located strictly in the varnish. These are considered by many authors as pathognomonic lesions for teeth in occlusal trauma [13,14]. These lesions with lack of dental hard tissues are located on the vestibular side. The section looks like an obtuse angle open to the mouth vestibule. The lesion affects hard coronary tissues but extends to the root cementum, in the same time with marginal periodontal retraction [5,15,16]. The color of the cuneiform lesions walls is slightly modified and they have a hard consistency, heat sensitivity or chemical is inconsistent and injury has a slow progress. If you are creating a five grade cavity lesion evolves rapidly while getting the characteristics of dental cavity. Occlusal obstacles and / or occlusal parafunctions often cause appearance of pathological abrasion [13]. It should be clinically noted how the abrasion is dependent on other factors. It is demonstrates that the patient's age, degree of abrasion of tooth of specific subject, the presence of eccentric abrasion (which betrays occlusion function) are factors that cause pathological abrasion [4].

Studies show that reducing the masticatory field by edentation accelerates abrasion. Local hyperacidity (by diet or acid regurgitation) can lead to erosion (as opposed to abrasion) [17]. Presence of enamel dystrophy and dysplasia, in one word the quality of dental hard tissues is an important factor that causes tooth wear [18].Another extremely important factor that can cause tooth wear is the abrasive capacity of prosthetic restoration materials.Isolated clinical examination makes it virtually impossible to determine the rate of pathological abrasion. Therefore it is prudent that in such cases to make exploratory therapeutic methods (selective grinding, temporary dentures) before major restaurateurs interventions. In this way, the dentist is able to identify more precisely the primary determinant of pathological abrasion and abrasion evolution speed.General pathological abrasion-is the abrasion inconsistent with biological age. The generalized pathological abrasion is a major sign of dysfunctional occlusal [18,19].

Periodontal pockets do not occur in primary occlusal trauma, but usually in secondary, on a periodontium already affected in the presence of infectious and local irritative factors. As long as the inflammation is limited to the gum, it is not aggravated by traumatic occlusal forces, but when the inflammatory process spreads to desmodontium own tissue, the occlusal trauma becomes a co-destruction factor of support structures, protecting the periodontal pockets of bones. A periodontal pockets is pathological deepening of the gingivodental fosse which is formed gradually, resulting the destruction of tooth support tissue and its mobility, finally leading to its expulsion of [19].

Destructive alveolar processes represent another consequence of the occlusal trauma phenomenon. Alveolar bone, despite of its appearance rigidity, is less stable than periodontal tissue, as is continuous-changing structure by obvious resorption phenomenon in the pressure area and by apposition ones manifested within traction territory. In the case of occlusal trauma, the destructive effect on alveolar bone is directly proportional to the overload degree, their frequency and duration being inversely proportional to the resistance of the tissue. On such a field, under the action of repeated occlusion constraints, the negative effects of occlusal trauma occur more easily, periodontal disease having a fast and serious evolution. In conjunction of any occlusal trauma caused by bruxism amid a normal gum, first the bone destruction presents the characteristic of an aseptic process, lytic, of some areas that cannot be radiologically detected yet. In later stages, due to parafunction persistence, destructive phenomena complicate, the blood nutrition being even more deficient, due to prolonged action of pressure forces, amid local irritations (tartar and plaque) will contribute to the failure of the epithelial barrier to invasion of microorganisms and toxins. The existing bone bags, along with the gum ones installed will progress simultaneously, adding also the gingival retraction [20]. Another result of the occlusion dysfunction is represented by the opening of the interproximal contacts. The consequence of periodontal changes caused by occlusal trauma is represented by dental mobility, dental migrations, and gingivorragia. Mobility is due to an occlusal trauma exerted on that tooth, the tooth receiving abnormal forces which pressure it during protrusion and laterotrusion movements.

The more frequently there are affected the monoradiculars that are subjected to occlusal trauma producing bone lysis in the support periodontium level. Because of dental mobility is difficult to detect when occlusal trauma occurs, requiring consideration of occlusion, both in centric relation and maximum intercuspation and also in protrusion and laterotrusion movements. Pathological tooth migration is a phenomenon that occurs due to poor periodontal structure, exacerbating existing traumatic occlusion with more pronounced effect of paraxial transmission of masticatory forces so harmful to the entire dento-maxillary system. Changing the position of one or more teeth causes 'contact rupture' between them, creating spaces (trema, diastema) favoring mechanical injury of epithelial insertion with papilla inflammation often accompanied by bleeding. Implantation of the pluriradiculars is more favorable for the capacity of trauma resistance when the roots are divergent. In fact, all aspects mentioned above influence the capacity of occlusal trauma resistance, making a normal request to appear as supraliminal, emphasizing the traumatogenic character of occlusal forces [3, 21].

Coating or superficial periodontium injuries take various clinical forms depending on the intensity, duration and direction on which occlusal trauma manifests. Occlusal trauma can cause a progressive denudation of teeth roots, characterized by moving the gum to the tooth apex. There are two sets of gum retractions: one which is detected on physical examination, another one hidden, and a part of the root being covered by the inflamed wall of a periodontal pocket. It should be noted that gingival retraction may involve all insertion area from the level of dental package, or only partially. The most common areas are the vestibular and oral of one tooth, of a group of teeth or even of a complete dental arch.

Traumatic dental hygiene habits can worsen the gingival recessions at the level of vestibular teeth face, this being associated with the occurrence and emphasis of cuneiform injuries, which is a pathognomonic sign that the tooth / teeth in question are in occlusal trauma [22].

Occlusal trauma causes and aggravates the gingival retraction, thus accelerating the initial epithelial proliferation by a local irritation, clinical form known as Mc Call's garlands or festoons. It also can reveal injuries as cracks (Stillman's fissures). These identities are pathological bag bottoms in which the ulcerative process developed, they could spontaneously cicatrize or persist in the form of deep fissures with rolled edges [23, 24, 25]. Papilla and gingivitis occurring as a result of opening the cervical interproximal space arise as a consequence of the loss of dental contact points in the presence of partial edentation which are accompanied by migrations, tipping or translations of the limiting dental units to edentulous breaches. The opening of interproximal space allows food particles penetration, thus injuring the gingival papillae.

Local examination reveals the presence of gingival inflammation that may be associated with bleeding. In advanced stages there is a junction of the vestibular and oral gums, accompanied by a slight extrusion of the affected tooth. Interradicular space dissection is characterized by roots denudation, gingival epithelium covering the limbus bone top retreating. Reaching bifurcation or trifurcation root is generally due to deepening of vestibular gingivodental or oral channel [26, 27].

Any indiscriminate therapeutic act in terms of ignorance or underestimation the capacity features and adaptive limit capacity, respectively of teeth defense, periodontium, temporomandibular joint, jaw bones, neuromuscular and vascular complexes, is likely to confuse the morphofunctional balance of dento-maxillary system, thus prejudicing the treated subject through iatrogenesis.

2.2. Malocclusions

The interrelation between the periodontal health status, the presence of dento-maxillary anomalies and the orthodontic treatment remains a controversial issue in the literature [28], reflected in the great diversity of the findings of studies that address this issue. Some researchers promote the idea that the presence of dento-maxillary anomalies is a risk factor in the development of periodontal pathology: [29-34];

The dento-maxillary anomalies may represent a risk factor in producing chronic marginal periodontitis as they maintain the periodontal inflammation, while changing the intensity and direction of occlusal forces. Other periodontal changes as insufficient attached gingiva width and low height of the alveolar bone were also observed and associated with the presence of dento-maxillary anomalies in general, or a single misaligned teeth [35, 36], as well as people with evident dento-maxillary anomalies were discovered to whom periodontal changes were minimal or nonexistent [37].

2.2.1. Dento-alveolar disharmony (DAD) with crowding

They are a risk factor for the presence of septic inflammation, because due to the disparity between mesial-distal sizes of permanent teeth and corresponding alveolar arches' perimeter, various dental malposition occur, localized mainly in incisor-canine region (Figure 1), which causes retention of food debris and plaque, and difficulty in removing them by self-cleaning or artificial cleaning [38]. This correlation is weaker in the maxilla compared to the mandible [39].

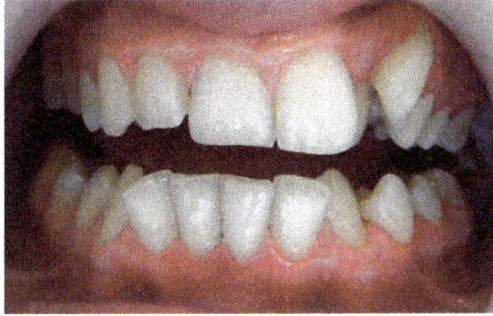

Figure 1. Gingival inflammation with papillae hypertrophy in lower and upper incisors, thin periodontium at 23 (eruption in buccal position) in a patient with dental crowding

The fact that malocclusion with crowding is a risk factor in the development of periodontal pathology is supported by studies that have reported the existence of a strong correlation between the presence of this anomaly and the occurrence of periodontal pockets, [40]; [41]; or the reduction of alveolar bone[42].

Anatomical conditions specific to this anomaly are unfavorable because interdental septa are thin, interdental papillae are laminated, with low volume and with poor blood circulation, unfavorable for a good gingival-periodontal nutrition [43].

2.2.2. Dento-alveolar disharmony (DAD) with spacing

DAD cause periodontal adaptive phenomena such as: hiperkeratinized epithelium, gingival chorion fibrosis, flattening dental papilla (which become a plateau or even concave aspect) (Figure 2). The presence of this anomaly may favor direct trauma on interdental papillae by food fragments.

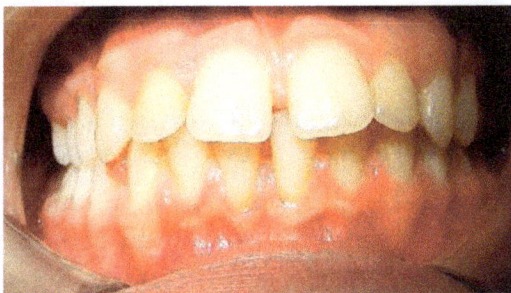

Figure 2. Gingival retractions with a thin periodontium at 31, 41, aplatized papillae between 11 and 21

Many specialized studies could not establish any positive correlation between incongruence with spacing and periodontal parameters in conditions of a rigorous hygiene, so that there are authors who consider that the indication for closure of interdental spaces is aesthetic rather than for periodontal dental health maintaining. [39]

2.2.3. Open bite

In the anterior open bite teeth are not functionaly requested during mastication (missing the food cut), and the self-cleaning phenomenon is absent favoring installation of gingival inflammation and hyperplastic changes. In contrast, lateral teeth are in occlusal contact and they are overworked during masticatory effort, they being almost in a state of permanent occlusal trauma due to the transfer of mandibular movements' previous guide of the lateral teeth [44].

We thus witness the periodontal space widening, gingival retraction emergence and horizontal bone atrophy of these teeth.

According to Macht and Zubery [45], in this syndrome we are witnessing a significant increase in the gingival inflammation, consequence of the enhancing virulence of the dehydrated plaque (due to lack of labial competence), and an increase in the length of the clinical crowns of incisors, which may suggest that open bite predisposes patients to the development of gingival retractions localized in the incisor segment (Figure 3).

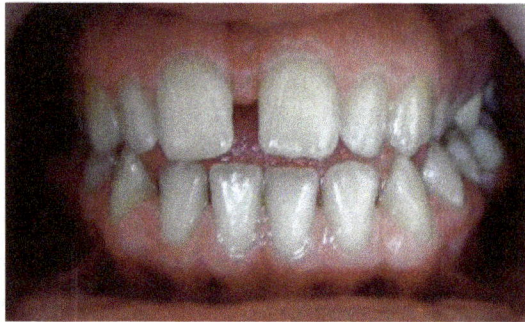

Figure 3. Open bite in a 19 years patient-thin periodontium predisposed at gingival recessions

2.2.4. Deep bite (class II division 2 malocclusion)

In the deep bite syndrome, anterior teeth don't have stable occlusal stops, and their implantation remains normal just as long as inflammation isn't installed due to the presence of plaque. When gingival-periodontal injuries of microbial cause occur, the anterior teeth implantation degrades, it begins a process of accelerated active eruption of the anterior inferior teeth, with the possibility of their direct trauma to the incisive upper periodontium [43], and the progression of periodontal lesions. Deep bite syndrome will lead in these conditions to increased periodontal pocket depth and marginal gingival retractions appearance [39]

2.2.5. Overbite (class II division 1 malocclusions)

Due to inocclusion lips and upper lip hypotrophy, bacterial accumulation occurs in the anterior dental area, the immunological role of saliva is reduced, and on long-term increases the frequency of periodontal lesions [46]. Similar to open bite, in the anterior dental regions, a fragile periodontal can be structured (Figure 4), prone to periodontal lesions because of unstable interdental contacts. The same fragile periodontium can be observed in the side areas, due to unilateral or bilateral crossbite (consequences of a different degree of compression of the two jaws).

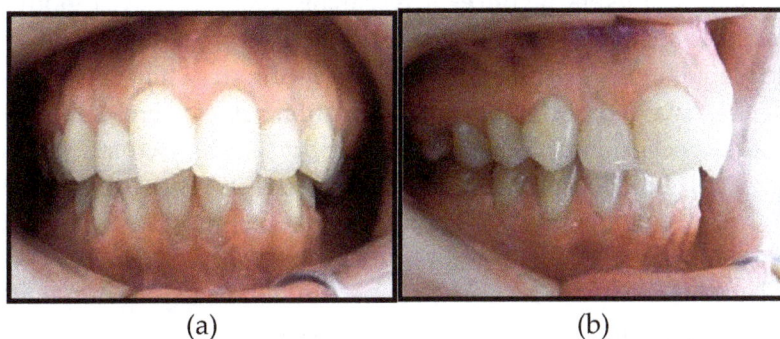

(a)   (b)

Figure 4. Fragile periodontium with gingival recessions in lower incisors (a-frontal b-lateral view) in a patient with maxillary compression

There is no concordance of views regarding correlations between sagittal inocclusion (overjet) and periodontal parameters. Authors such as Davies et al. 1991, [47] or Geiger et al., 1976, [48] support the existence of a significant correlation between plaque index, periodontal diseases and severe anterior overjet (> 6 mm), while Buckley, 1981 [49] considers that there is no significant correlation between the presence of overjet and plaque index, or gingival inflammation index.

According to Torres et al., 2006, [50] an increase in the plaque index occurs only in subjects with sagittal inocclusion > 6, and after Bjornaas et al. 1994 [51], to adulthood, in the presence of a severe sagittal inocclusion (overjet ≥8mm), there is a reduction of alveolar bone level with ≈0,96mm in the upper anterior area, and with ≈0,35 mm in the lower area.

2.2.6. Mandibular prognathism (class III malocclusions)

In mandibular prognathism, the lingual pressure (of the protrude tongue and low positioned) continuously exercised on the lower incisors' lingual face and the occlusal trauma due to anterior crossbite can lead to important vestibulo-version of the mandibular incisors with fine periodontal biotypes inducing and the presence of a very thin vestibular cortical bone, located away from the cemento-enamel junction.

Transferring anterior guide on the lateral teeth, found in this group of anomalies, leads to the lateral dental area overloading concurrent to a less loading of the front area (no food incision)

[44]. Therefore we can expect the emergence of periodontal changes like horizontal bone atrophy and epithelial insertion's descent [52].

Periodontal changes occur early in reverse gear and consist of the occurrence of significant gingival retraction of the lower incisors' vestibular face ("disposal trench"), possibly a tooth mobility, following a permanent occlusal trauma.

These periodontal changes can regress spontaneously if orthodontic treatment is instituted early [53].

There is no uniformity of opinion or about the association between anterior crossbite with different periodontal parameters. Ngom et al. researches 2005, [39] have reported the presence of a significant correlation between anterior crossbite and the percentage of gingival retraction, but not with the plaque index and the gingival pockets depth, while Hashim and Al-Jasser's researches, 1996, [54] have found a significant correlation between crossbite, the plaque index and the periodontal pocket depth. The difference between the two studies may be due to differences in age and dental hygiene of the subjects investigated. Silness and Roynstrand, 1984, [55] opines that the crossbite teeth show more frequently signs of periodontal disease compared to those dealing a normal occlusion.

2.2.7. Congenital malformations of the lip, maxilla and palate(clefts)

Next to specific anatomical defects, the delays in the formation and timing of tooth eruption, the need for long orthodontic treatment [56, 57] and the presence of prosthetic restorations are factors contributing to the reduction of the alveolar bone level in areas adjacent to dehiscence [58].

Multiple dental malposition, segmental alveolar gaps, soft tissue folds made before palatoplasty, the presence of scar tissue or oro-nasal communications persisting after surgical closure of the defect, make oral hygiene maintenance a difficult task, increasing risk and progression of periodontal disease [59, 60, 61].

Comparing the periodontium from patients with cleft lip and cleft palate, to the one from patients with cleft palate only, Gaggl et al., 1999, [62 found that the first have a predisposition to deep periodontal destructions in the teeth adjacent to the splicing area, while in patients that only have cleft palate, clinical peridental appearance may be similar to that of subjects without malformations. However, Dewinter and Quirynen state that the periodontium of the teeth from the splicing zone or near it, in patients with unilateral cleft, can cope relatively well to a long orthodontic treatment or to a combined periodontal-orthodontic treatment [63].

2.3. Orthodontic treatment

The three main reasons justifying the need for orthodontic treatment are: to improve facial and dental aesthetics, oro-dental health and the normal oral functions [36].

In the absence of periodontal diseases and in the presence of a proper oral hygiene, a well led orthodontic treatment should not have, on long-term, significant effects on periodontal supportive structures. According to Graber et al., 2005, [64] it is possible to occur a decrease in the alveolar bone's volume and height, as an adaptive process to the trauma.

The main clinical periodontal effects that can be seen in the oral cavity after insertion of orthodontic appliances are: gingival hyperplasia, marginal gingival retraction, irreversible loss of bone support and excessive fibrous tissue that prevents complete closure of the post extraction spaces [65].

2.3.1. Gingival overgrowth (hypertrophy and hyperplasia)

A periodontal change frequently observed during orthodontic treatment, especially with fixed appliances, is the emergence of gingival overgrowth [66].

Scope, they can be localized or generalized, but seem to be more common in mandibular incisors region (67, 68) (Figure 5).

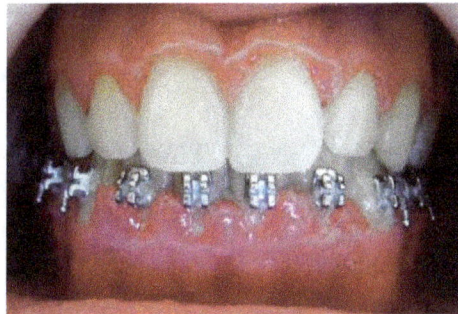

Figure 5. Gingival overgrowth with inflammation and plaque accumulation in the lower incisors

Other authors (69) believe that overgrowths may be marginal, diffuse, papillary, or discrete and have four degrees of severity:

• 0-no gingival overgrowth;

• I – gingival overgrowth extended only to the dental papilla;

• II-gingival overgrowth covering the papilla and marginal gingiva;

• III-gingival overgrowth covers three quarters or more of the dental crown.

Since gingival overgrowth is a factor limiting or preventing orthodontic tooth movement, it often requires its removal by gingivectomy, which removes all fibrous tissues around the tooth and at the same time allows gum's reshaping or remodeling [69]. After gingivectomy, periodontal condition is improving, so the orthodontic mechanic's normal course is possible. If it does not prevent the effectiveness of orthodontic treatment and causes no discomfort to the patient, gum volume enlargement can be removed after the completion of orthodontic treatment, if it does not regress spontaneously.

2.3.2. Marginal gingival retractions and losses of bone support

Sometimes, the incidence of gingival recessions in patients with a fixed orthodontic appliance can be up to 10% [70]. In addition, repeated trauma on marginal gingiva by teeth movements and plaque accumulation, inherent with the application of orthodontic appliances, can lead to the formation of marginal gingival retractions. Moreover, mucogingival problems prior to the initiation of orthodontic treatment could be exacerbated by the application of orthodontic force [70]. It seems that the lower incisors are the teeth most likely to develop marginal gingival retractions, the mechanism of their occurrence being the excessive force applying, which does not allow bone's repairing or remodeling during teeth movement with the existence of a thin or non-existent vestibular cortical and an inadequate or absent keratinized gum [40].

2.3.3. Assesment of periodontal changes using immunological analysis in Gingival Crevicular Fluid (GCF)

During the initial phase of orthodontic treatment, orthodontic forces induce a response to the mechanical stress from periodontium and a net of events it is produced: angiogenesis, aseptic inflammation and periodontal remodeling [71].

Gingival crevicular fluid (GCF) is used to determine the presence and levels of biomarkers expressed during the first phase of orthodontic treatment, this cascade of substances comprising cytokines, metalloproteinases and other mediators of complex transformations in the periodontium [72, 73].

In studies funded by the grant ID573/2008 of the Ministry of Education and Research of Romania, we measured the levels of Pentraxin-3 (PTX3), Thrombospondin1 (TSP1), Lipocalin2/Matrix metalloproteinase 9 (MMP9/NGAL) complex and Matrix metalloproteinase 9 (MMP9) in GCF at different time points of the first 2 weeks of orthodontic treatment, to determine the relationship between these values and theirs implication in inflammation and angiogenesis balance, in the situation of a good control of the bacterial plaque [74, 75].

GCF samples were collected from orthodontic patients requiring upper canine distalization with first premolar extraction. For the orthodontic appliance, there are placed brackets Roth 0.018 inch (GAC Intl, Bohemia, USA) with 0.012 inch NiTi archwire (GAC Intl, Bohemia, USA) and a laceback made from 0.010 inch stainless wire, placed and activated 21 days after the premolar extraction.

Using the statistical analysis, our results show a change in time of PTX3, TSP1, MMP9/NGAL and MMP9 levels in GCF of patients with this method of orthodontic treatment and suggest their stronger involvement in inflammation and angiogenesis processes in PDL during orthodontic periodontal remodeling, in the situation of a healthy periodontium and a good control of the bacterial plaque.

2.3.4. Assessment of periodontal changes using immunohistochemical analysis of gingival tissue

The gingival overgrowth as a reaction of the orthodontic treatment was longtime considered by the clinicians as an inflammatory result of the retention of the bacterial plaque by the orthodontic devices. Clinical observations showed that the gingival overgrowth appear also in patients with good oral hygiene, without any clinical signs of gingival inflammation.

Our studies [76,77] in the grant ID573/2008 funded by the Ministry of Education and Research in Romania showed that the gingival overgrowth during the fixed orthodontic treatment appears at the beginning, without any inflammatory signs, as a result of the mechanical stress and periodontal remodeling during the orthodontic movement, the MMP8 and MMP9 acting as indicators of this situation.The inflammation of gingiva occurs as a consequence of the accumulation of the bacterial plaque favorized by the orthodontic devices.

Gingivectomy was performed in patient with gingival overgrowth in the first eight weeks of the orthodontic treatment and the material obtained was used for histologic and immunohistochemical study.

3. Systemic factors and periodontal changes

3.1. Diabetes and obesity

Diabetes mellitus (DM) and periodontitis are both chronic inflammatory disorders and which enhances their severity, worsen each other prognosis and share a number of pathogenic mechanisms with common inflammatory mediators which have been investigated as possible biomarkers of disease status.These improved diagnostic efforts resulting from utilization of biomarkers should enable optimal treatment planning, also assist in monitoring clinical response to treatment and more focused prevention of common human conditions. The most important inflammatory mediators linked to initiation and progression of periodontal disease is a complex network of pro-inflammatory cytokines, matrix metalloproteinases (MMPs) and prostaglandins [78]. The vast majority of studies of cytokines, adipokines and other mediators in periodontitis and diabetes have been small-scale clinical studies using GCF(gingival crevicular fluid), saliva or gingival tissues samples which have focused on limited number of mediators and many inconclusive because of limitation in study design. Nevertheless there are promising data on certain mediators such IL-1β, IL-6, TNF-α and emerging data on RANKL and OPG; these are likely to have a central role in the pathogenesis of periodontitis in diabetic patients [79, 80]. Complex interactions between individual mediators and emergent pathways, for example, synergy in cytokine signaling, will not be apparent from simple disease association studies of a limited number of molecules [79, 80].

There are studies suggesting that pro-inflammatory cytokines which induce chronic inflammatory diseases including periodontitis, could increase insulin resistance [81, 82]. Both TNF-α and IL-6 are produced in adipose tissue, and a large quantity of circulating IL-6 is derived [83]. There are also studies which correlate periodontitis to obesity [84, 85]. These directions of research suggest that obesity, diabetes and periodontitis may be related to each other.

Effective periodontal treatment in patients with DM significantly reduced GCF [86, 87] and serum levels of several mediators, such as IL6, TNF, adiponectin [88, 89, 90], MMP2, MMP9 [91], thus leading to reduced systemic inflammation.

In the effort to establish a pathway for the periodontitis-DM-obesity co-morbidity, some studies have determined genetic polymorphisms for IL6 and IL1 [92, 93]. These cytokines have been previously measured in blood and GFC from patients with these diseases.

Because fatty tissue serves as a reservoir for inflammatory cytokines, an increase in body fat may determine an increase of the inflammatory response of the host in periodontal disease [94].

In 2014, a study concerning the low fibers rich and fat poor diet for 8 weeks, demonstrated an improvement of the periodontal disease's markers, their levels returning to the initial value after follow-up period [95]. A study proposed the hyperinflammatory state observed in obesity, determined by the increase in cytokine levels, as mechanism to explain this relation [96].

Aknowledgment

Immunological and immunohistochemical studies of MMP9/NGAL, TSP1, PTX3, MMP8 and MMP9 in GCF and gingival tissue of orthodontic patients were funded by the grant ID573/2008 of the Ministry of Education and Research of Romania, IDEAS competition of CNCSIS.

Author details

Petra Surlin[1], Anne Marie Rauten[2], Mihai Raul Popescu[3], Constantin Daguci[4] and Maria Bogdan[5]

1 University of Medicine and Pharmacy of Craiova, Faculty of Dental Medicine, Department of Periodontology, Romania

2 University of Medicine and Pharmacy of Craiova, Faculty of Dental Medicine, Department of Orthodontics, Romania

3 University of Medicine and Pharmacy of Craiova, Faculty of Dental Medicine, Department of Occlusal Sciences, Romania

4 University of Medicine and Pharmacy of Craiova, Faculty of Dental Medicine, Department of Oral Health, Romania

5 University of Medicine and Pharmacy of Craiova, Faculty of Pharmacy, Department of Pharmacology, Romania

References

[1] ASH. Dental Anatomy Phisiology and Occlusion. W. B. Saunders Co.1993; 45-68,89-146.

[2]   Gray HS. Occlusion and restorative dentistry: Part1.NZDent J1993; 89(395):61-5.

[3]   Calandriello M, Carnevale G, Ricci G. Parodontologia, Ed. Martina Bologna 1996; 20-45,156-193,549-587.

[4]   Dawson PE. Position paper regarding diagnosis, management, and treatment of temporomandibular disorders. The American Equilibration Society. J Prosth Dent 1999; 81(2):174-8.

[5]   Lund JP Occlusion: the "science-based" approach. J Can Dent Assoc 2001; 67(2):84.

[6]   Millstein P, Maya A. An evaluation of occlusal contact marking indicators. A descriptive quantitative method. J Am Dent Ass 2001; 132(9):1280-6; quiz 1319.

[7]   Gremillion HA. The relationship beetwen occlusion and TMJ: an evidence-based discussion. J Evid Based Dent Pract 2006; 6:43-47.

[8]   Genco RJ. Current view of risk factors for periodontal diseases. J Periodontol 1996 Oct; 67(10 Suppl):1041-9.

[9]   Armitage GC. Periodontal diagnoses and classification of periodontal diseases. Periodontology 2004; 34:9-21.

[10] Harrel SK, Nunn ME, Hallmon WW. Is there an association betwen occlusion and periodontal destruction? Yes-occlusal forces can contribute to periodontal destruction. J Am Dent Assoc 2006; 137:1380-1384.

[11] Greenstein G, Greenstein B, Cavallaro J. Prerequisite for treatment planning implant dentistry: periodontal prognostication of compromised teeth. Compend Contin Educ Dent 2007; 28:436-437.

[12] MC Neill C. Occlusion: what it is and what it is not. J Calif Dent Assoc 2000; 28(10): 748-58.

[13] Dale R. Occlusion: the standard of care. J Can Dent Assoc 2003; 67(2):83-92.

[14] Telles D, Pegoraro LF, Pereira JC, et al. Incidence of noncarios cervical lesions and their relation to the presence of wear facets. J Esthet Restor Dent 2006; 18: 178-183.

[15] Grippo JO, Simring M, Schreiner S. Attrition, abrasion, corrosion and abfraction revisited: a new perspective on tooth surface lesions. J AM Dent Assoc 2004; 135:1109-1118

[16] Abrahamsen TC, The worn dentition-pathognomonic patterns of abrasion and erosion. Int Dent J 2005; 55:268-276.

[17] Coleman TA, Grippo JO, Kinderknecht KE. Cervical dentin hypersensitivity, Part III: resolution following occlusal equilibration. Quintessence Int 2003; 34:427-434.

[18] Dawson PE. Functional occlusion: from TMJ to Smile Design. St. Louis 2007:27-32.

[19] Ruiz Jl. Achieving Longevity in esthetic dentistry by proper diagnosis and management of occlusal disease. Contemporary Esthetics 2007;11:24-27.

[20] Williams Dm, Hughes FJ, Osell Ew, Farthing PM. Pathology of Periodontal Disease. Oxford University Press, 1992.

[21] Williams RC. Periodontal disease. N Engl J Med 1990; 8:322: 373-82

[22] Papapanou PN. Periodontal Disease: epidemiology. Ann Periodontol 1996; 1(1):1-36.

[23] Okesson J.P. Management of Temporomandibular Disorders and Occlusion, St. Louis, Mosby1993; 111, 125, 569;

[24] Armitage GC. Development of a classification system for periodontal diseases and conditions. Ann Perio 1999; 4:1-6.

[25] Avery JC. Oral development and hystology. Third edition, Ed. Thieme, Stuttgart, 2002.

[26] Wilson TG, Kornman KS. Fundamentals of Periodontics. Quintessence Publishing Co. Chicago, 1996

[27] Zaslansky P, Friesam AA, Weiner S. Structure and mechsnical properties of the soft zone separating bulk dentin and enamel in crown of human teeth. J Struct Biol 2006; 153:188-99.

[28] Johal A, Katsaros C, Kiliaridis S, Leitao P, Rosa M, Sculean A, Weiland F, Zachrisson B. State of the science on controversial topics: orthodontic therapy and gingival recession (a report of the Angle Society of Europe 2013 meeting). In: Johal et al. Progress in Orthodontics 2013;14-16.

[29] Helm S, Petersen PE. Causal relation between malocclusion and periodontal health. Acta Odontol Scand 1989 ;47(4):223-228.

[30] Abu Alhaija ES, Al-Wahadni AM. Relationship between tooth irregularity and periodontal disease in children with regular dental visits. J Clin Pediatr Dent 2006; 30(4): 296-8.

[31] Pugaca Jolanta, Urtane Ilga, Liepa Andra, Laurina Z. The relationship between the severity of malposition of the frontal teeth and periodontal health in age 15-21 and 35-44. Stomat Baltic Dent Maxillofac J 2007;9:86-90.

[32] Mtaya M, Brudvik P, Åstrøm AN. Prevalence of malocclusion and its relationship with socio-demographic factors, dental caries, and oral hygiene in 12-to 14-year-old Tanzanian schoolchildren. European Journal of Orthodontics 2009;31(5):467–476.

[33] Chandrasekhara Reddy V., Ashok Kumar BR., Ankola Anil. Relationship Between Gingivitis and Anterior Teeth Irregularities Among 18 to 26 Years Age Group: A Hospital Based Study in Belgaum, Karnataka. JOHCD 2010;4(3):61-66.

[34] Gusmão S Estela, Coutinho de Queiroz RD, de Souza Coelho Renata, Cimões Renata, Lima dos Santos Rosenês. Association between malpositioned teeth and periodontal disease. Dental Press J Orthod 2011;16(4):87-94

[35] Bimstein, E., Needleman, H.L., Karimbux, N., Van Dyke, T.E. Malocclusion, orthodontic intervention, and gingival and periodontal health-Periodontal and Gingival Health and Diseases – Children, Adolescents, and Yong Adults. Ed Martin Dunity 2001;17-31, 251-273.

[36] Ngom P.I, Benoist, H.M., Thiam, F., Diagne, F., Diallo, P.D. Influence of orthodontic anomalies on periodontal condition. Odontostomatol Tropic 2007;30(118):9-16.

[37] Onyeaso, C.O., Arowojolu, M.O., Taiwo, J.O. Periodontal status of orthodontic patients and the relationship between dental aesthetic index and community periodontal index of treatment need. Am J Orthod Dentofacial Orthop 2003;124(6):714-20

[38] Ashley FP, Usiskin LA, Wilson RF, Wagaiyu E. The relationship between irregularity of the incisor teeth, plaque, and gingivitis: a study in a group of schoolchildren aged 11-14 years. Eur J Orthop 1998;20:65-72.

[39] Ngom PI, Benoist, H.M., Thiam, F., Diagne, F., Diallo, P.D. Intraarch and interarch relationships of the anterior teeth and periodontal conditions. Angle Orthod 2005;76(2):236-242.

[40] EL-Mangoury NH, Gaafar SM, Mostafa YA. Mandibular anterior crowding and periodontal disease. Angle Orthod 1987;1:33-38.

[41] Staufer K, Landmesser H. Effects of crowding in the lower anterior segment—a risk evaluation depending upon the degree of crowding. J Orofac Orthop 2004;65:13-25.

[42] Jensen L, Birgit, Solow B. Alveolar bone loss and crowding in adult periodontal patients. Community Dent Oral Epidemiol 1989;17(1):47–51.

[43] Dumitiu HT. *Parodontologie*. Ed Viaţa Medical Rom 1998;92-94

[44] Dorobăţ Valentina, Stanciu D. Ortodonţie şi ortopedie dento-facială. Ed Med 2009:363-457.

[45] Machtei EE, Zubery Y, Bimstein E, Becker A. Anterior open bite and gingival recession in children and adolescents. Int Dent J, 1990;40(6):369-373.

[46] Bassigny F. Manuel d'orthopedie dento-faciale. Paris: Masson: 1991.

[47] Davies TM, Shaw WC, Worthington HV, Addy M, Dummer P, Kingdon A. The effect of orthodontic treatment on plaque and gingivitis. Am J Orthod Dentofac Orthop 1991;99:155-161.

[48] Geiger AM, Wasserman BH. Relationship of occlusion and periodontal disease: part IX. Incisor inclination and periodontal status. Angle Orthod 1976;46(2):99-110.

[49] Buckley LA. The relationships between irregular teeth, plaque, calculus and gingival disease. A study of 300 subjects. British Dental Journal 1980:148(3):67-69.

[50] Torres H., Corrêa S. Daniela, Zenóbio EG. Avaliação da condição periodontal em pacientes de 10 a 18 anos com diferentes más oclusões. R Dental Press Ortodon Ortop Facial 2006;11(6):73-80.

[51] Bjornaas T, Rygh P, Boe OE. Severe overjet and overbite reduced alveolar bone height in 19-year-old men. Am J Orthod Dentofacial Orthop 1994;106(2):139-45.

[52] Glăvan Florica, Jianu Rodica. Ortodonţie. Ed Miron 1999;229

[53] Boboc G. Anomaliile dento-maxilare. Ed Medicală, Bucureşti, 1971;9-146.

[54] Hashim HA, Al-Jasser NM. Periodontal findings in cases of posterior cross-bite. J Clin Pediatr Dent 1996;20:317-320.

[55] Silness J, Roynstrand T. Effects on dental health of spacing of teeth in anterior segments. J Clin Periodontol 1984;11:387-398.

[56] Lages EM., Marcus B., Pordeus IA. Oral health of individuals with cleft lip, cleft palate, or both. Cleft Palate Craniofac J 2004;41:59-63.

[57] Quirynen M., Dewinter G., Avontoodt P., Heidbuchel K., Verdonck A., Carels C. A split mouth study on periodontal and microbiological parameters in children with complete unilateral cleft lip and palate. J Clin Periodontol 2003;30:49-56.

[58] Stec Magdalena, Szczepańska Joanna, Pypeć J., Hirschfelder Ursula. Periodontal Status and Oral Hygiene in Two Populations of Cleft Patients. The Cleft Palate-Craniofac J 2007;44(1):73-78.

[59] Boloor V., Thomas B. Comparison of periodontal status among patients with cleft lip, cleft palate, and cleft lip along with a cleft in palate and alveolus. J Indian Soc Periodontol 2010;14(3):168-172.

[60] Costa B., Lima JE., Gomide MR., Rosa OP. Clinical and microbiological evaluation of the periodontal status of children with unilateral complete cleft lip and palate. Cleft Palate Craniofac J 2003;40:585–589.

[61] Wong F., King N. The oral health of children with clefts: a review. Cleft Palate-Craniofac J 1998;35:248-254.

[62] Gaggl A, Schultes G, Kärcher H, Mossböck R. Periodontal disease in patients with cleft palate and patients with unilateral and bilateral clefts of lip, palate and alveolus. J Periodontol 1999;70(2):171-8.

[63] Dewinter G, Quirynen M, Heidbüchel K, Verdonck A, Willems G, Carels C. Dental abnormalities, bone graft quality and periodontal conditions in patients with unilateral cleft lip and palate at different phases of orthodontic treatment. Cleft Palate Cranoifacial J 2003;40(4):343-50.

[64] Graber TM., Vanarsdall RL., Vig KW. Orthodontics-Current Principles and Techniques-5th ed. St Louis, Elsevier Mosby, 2012; 807-842.

[65] Krishnan V, Ambili R, Davidovitch Z, Murphy NC. Gingiva and Orthodontic Treatment. Semin Orthod 2007;13:257-271.

[66] Kouraki E., Bissada NF., Palomo JM., Ficara AJ. Gingival enlargement and resolution during and after orthodontic therapy. N Y State Dent J 2005;71(4):34-37.

[67] Zachrisson BU., Alnaes L. Periodontal condition in orthodontically treated and untreated individuals-I. Loss of attachment, gingival pocket depth and clinical crown height. Angle Orthod 1973;43:402-411.

[68] Zachrisson S., Zachrisson BU. Gingival condition associated with orthodontic treatment. Angle Orthod 1972;42:26-34.

[69] Newman MG., Takei HH., Klokkevold PR., Caranzza F. Carranza's Clinical Periodontology-9th edition. W.B. Saunders Co, Philadelphia 2002;279-297.

[70] Geiger AM. Mucogingival problems and the movement of mandibular incisors-a clinical review. Am J Orthod 1980;78:511-527.

[71] V. Krishnan and Z. Davidovitch, "On a path to unfolding the biological mechanism of orthodontic tooth movement", Journal of Dental Research, vol.88, no. 7, pp. 597-609, 2009

[72] J. Jr. Capelli, A. Kantarci, A. Haffajee et al., "Matrix metalloproteinases and chemokines in gingival crevicular fluid during orthodontic tooth movement", European Journal of Orthodontics, vol. 33, no. 6, pp. 705-711, 2011

[73] M.M. Bildt , M. Bloemen , A.M. Kuijpers-Jagtman , J.W. Von den Hoff, "Matrix metalloproteinases and tissue inhibitors of metalloproteinases in gingival crevicular fluid during orthodontic tooth movement", European Journal of Orthodontics, vol. 31, no. 5, pp. 529-537, 2010.

[74] Surlin P, Rauten AM, Silosi I, Foia L. Pentraxin-3 levels in gingival crevicular fluid during orthodontic tooth movement in young and adult patients. Angle Orthod. 2012 Sep; 82(5):833-8. doi: 10.2319/072911-478.1. Epub 2012 Jan 3.

[75] Surlin P, Silosi I, Rauten AM, Cojocaru M, Foia L. Involvement of TSP1 and MMP9/ NGAL in angiogenesis during orthodontic periodontal remodeling. ScientificWorldJournal. 2014; 2014:421029. doi: 10.1155/2014/421029. Epub 2014 May 20.

[76] Surlin P, Rauten AM, Mogoantă L, Siloşi I, Oprea B, Pirici D. Correlations between the gingival crevicular fluid MMP8 levels and gingival overgrowth in patients with fixed orthodontic devices. Rom J Morphol Embryol. 2010; 51(3):515-9.

[77] Şurlin P, Rauten AM, Pirici D, Oprea B, Mogoantă L, Camen A. Collagen IV and MMP-9 expression in hypertrophic gingiva during orthodontic treatment. Rom J Morphol Embryol. 2012; 53(1):161-5.

[78] Hanes PJ, Krishna R Characteristics of inflammation common to both diabetes and periodontitis: are predictive diagnosis and targeted preventive measures possible? EPMA J. 2010 Mar; 1(1):101-16. doi: 10.1007/s13167-010-0016-3

[79] P.M. Preshaw, A.L. Alba, D.Herrera, S. Jepsen, A. Konstantinidis, K. Makrilakis, R. Taylor Periodontitis and diabetes: a two-way relationship. Diabetologia 2012; 55:21-31

[80] Taylor JJ, Preshaw PM, Lalla E. A review of the evidence for pathogenic mechanisms that may link periodontitis and diabetes. J Clin Periodontol 2013; 40 (Suppl. 14)

[81] Hotamisligil GS, Peraldi P, Budavari A, Ellis R, White MF, Spiegelman BM. IRS-1-mediated inhibition of insulin receptor tyrosine kinase activity in TNF-alpha-and obesity-induced insulin resistance. Science 1996; 271: 665-668.

[82] Uysal KT, Wiesbrock SM, Marino MW, Hotamisligil GS. Protection from obesity-induced insulin resistance in mice lacking TNFalpha function. Nature 1997; 389: 610-614.

[83] Mohamed-Ali V, Goodrick S, Rawesh A et al. Subcutaneous adipose tissue releases interleukin-6, but not tumor necrosis factoralpha, in vivo. J Clin Endocrinol Metab 1997; 82: 4196-4200.

[84] Franchini R, Petri A, Migliario M, Rimondini L Poor oral hygiene and gingivitis are associated with obesity and overweight status in paediatric subjects. J Clin Periodontol 2011; 38: 1021–1028

[85] Haffajee AD, Socransky SS. Relation of body mass index, periodontitis and Tannerella forsythia. J Clin Periodontol 2009; 36: 89–99.

[86] Duarte PM, Szeremeske de Miranda T, Lima JA, Dias Gonçalves, Expression of Immune-Inflammatory Markers in Sites of Chronic Periodontitis in Type 2 Diabetic Subjects. J Periodontol 2011; DOI:10.1902/jop.2011.110324

[87] Hardy DC, Ross JH, Schuyler CA, Leite RS, Matrix metalloproteinase-8 expression in periodontal tissues surgically removed from diabetic and non-diabetic patients with periodontal disease. J Clin Periodontol 2011; DOI: 10.1111/j.1600-051X.2011.01788.x

[88] Chen L, Luo G, Xuan D, Wei B, Liu F, Li J, Zhang J, Effects of Non-surgical Periodontal Treatment on Clinical Response, Serum Inflammatory Parameters, and Metabolic Control in Type 2 Diabetic Patients: A Randomized Study J Periodontol 2011; DOI: 10.1902/jop.2011.110327.

[89] Kardeşler L, Buduneli N, Çetinkalp S, Lappin D, Kinane DF, Gingival crevicular fluid IL-6, tPA, PAI-2, albumin levels following initial periodontal treatment in chronic periodontitis patients with or without type 2 diabetes. Inflamm Res 2011; 60(2): 143-51.

[90] Sun WL, Chen LL, Zhang SZ, Wu YM, Ren YZ, Qin GM, Inflammatory cytokines, adiponectin, insulin resistance and metabolic control after periodontal intervention

in patients with type 2 diabetes and chronic periodontitis. Intern Med 2011; 50(15): 1569-74.

[91] Panagiotis A Koromantzos, Konstantinos Makrilakis, Xanthippi Dereka, Steven Offenbacher, Nicholas Katsilambros, Effect of Non-Surgical Periodontal Therapy on CRP, Oxidative Stress, MMP-9 and MMP-2 Levels in Patients With Type 2 Diabetes. A Randomized Controlled Study J Periodontol DOI:10.1902/jop.2011.110148

[92] Xiao LM, Yan YX, Xie CJ, Fan WH, Xuan DY, Association among interleukin-6 gene polymorphism, diabetes and periodontitis in a Chinese population Oral Diseases 2009; 15(8):547–553.

[93] López NJ, Valenzuela CY, Jara L, Interleukin-1 gene cluster polymorphisms associated with periodontal disease in type 2 diabetes. J Periodontol 2009; 80(10):1590-8.

[94] Ritchie CS. Obesity and periodontal disease. Periodontol 2000 2007; 44: 154-63

[95] Kondo K, Ishikado A, Morino K, Nishio Y, Ugi S, Kajiwara S, Kurihara M,Iwakawa H, Nakao K, Uesaki S, Shigeta Y, Imanaka H, YoshizakiT, Sekine O, Makino T, Maegawa H, King GL, Kashiwagi A. A high fiber, low-fat diet improves periodontal disease markers in high-risk subjects: a pilot study. Nutr Res 2014 Jun; 34(6):491-8.

[96] Sophia S, Jaideep M. Multifactorial Relationship of Obesity and Periodontal Disease. J Clin Diagn Res Apr 2014; 8(4): ZE01–ZE03

3

Periodontal Health and Orthodontics

Mourad Sebbar, Zouhair Abidine,
Narjisse Laslami and Zakaria Bentahar

1. Introduction

The most common objectives of an orthodontic treatment are facial and dental aesthetics and the improvement in the masticatory function. There is a continuously increasing number of adult patients who actively seek orthodontic treatment, and it is also an undeniable fact that the incidence of periodontal disease increases with age. Therefore, the number of patients with periodontal problems that attend orthodontic practices is significantly greater than in the past [1].

There are many links between periodontology and orthodontics. After all, every orthodontic intervention has a periodontal dimension: orthodontic biomechanics and treatment planning are basically determined by periodontal factors such as the length and shape of the roots, the width and height of the alveolar bone, and the structure of the gingiva [2].

The main objective of periodontal therapy is to restore and maintain the health and integrity of the attachment apparatus of teeth. Additionally, orthodontic therapy can facilitate management of several restorative and aesthetic problems relating to fractured teeth, tipped abutment teeth, excess spacing, inadequate pontic space, malformed teeth, and diastema.

Generally, the main reasons routinely cited to justify the provision of orthodontic treatment are improvement of facial and dental aesthetics and of dental health and function. However, association between malocclusions and periodontal condition is still controversial [3].

Ngom [4] found significant correlations between malocclusions and periodontal condition and suggested that malocclusions are risk markers for periodontal diseases. However, a real inference about a cause/effect relationship between malocclusions and periodontal condition in this study was not possible.

A review of the literature conducted by Van Gastel [5] showed contradictory findings on the impact of malocclusion and orthodontic appliances on periodontal health, since only a few studies reported attachment loss during orthodontic treatment. It has been suggested that this contradiction may be partly due to the selection of materials and differences in the research methods employed [6].

All evidence-based literature concerning the orthodontic-periodontic relationships show that a good orthodontic treatment of patients, who have excellent oral hygiene and do not suffer any periodontal breakdown, is a non-harmful treatment for the periodontium, it has been also demonstrated that a diminished oral hygiene in corporation with periodontal disorder would make the orthodontic treatment a real high risk for the periodontium [7.8].

In the modern and serious dental practice, such synergy is fundamental. Besides systemic variables, genetic heritance, age, collaboration, correct and complete diagnosis and good execution, the factor that isexplicitly mentioned in the literature as a must for success of the orthodontic therapy and of the periodontal therapy is the patient adequate oral hygiene [9].

A multidisciplinary approach is often necessary to treat and prevent dental problems in patients. This chapter will address basic considerations for orthodontists as well as periodontists for successful outcome of various treatments. Several clinical cases will be presented to illustrate the orthodontic-periodontic relationships.

2. Orthodontic treatment and oral hygiene

A high standard of oral hygiene is essential for patients undergoing orthodontic treatment. Without good oral hygiene, plaque accumulates around the orthodontic appliance, causing gingivitis and, in some cases, periodontal breakdown. To avoid such problems, the orthodontist has a double obligation: to advise the patient about methods of plaque control and, at routine visits, to monitor the effectiveness of the oral-hygiene regime. However, despite receiving appropriate advice, many patients undergoing orthodontic treatment fail to maintain an adequate standard of plaque control. It is important that the orthodontist is able to communicate the importance of oral hygiene to motivate patients to maintain a satisfactory standard of oral hygiene during orthodontic treatment [10].

Before any orthodontic treatment an initial diagnosis and referral for treatment to control active periodontal disease is to be considered. Moreover, all general, dental and periodontal treatment should be completed before the orthodontic treatment. Once the orthodontic appliances are placed, the patients need to be instructed in how to manage the new oral environment and how to maintain the health of the dental and periodontal structures. The orthodontist has to provide the patient with initial brushing instructions with either a conventional toothbrush or a powered one when the appliances are first placed. However, if the orthodontists correctly advice their patients to follow proper oral hygiene instructions during the orthodontic treatment is still an opened question.

Manual tooth brushing, one of the oldest methods of plaque removal, remains the basis of oral hygiene and plaque control. It is often used as the standard or control against which other methods of plaque removal are assessed [10,11]. Instruction should emphasize the need to use sufficient pressure to remove plaque; a pressure sensitive toothbrush would be a valuable aid to patients undergoing orthodontic treatment.

Chlorhexidine mouthwashes, as an adjunct to tooth brushing, have been found effective in the control of gingival inflammation [12], although prolonged use may cause problems with staining as Chlorhexidine rinses can potentially stain the margins of composite restorations that cannot be easily removed. More recently, pre-brushing rinses have been introduced, though these show no differences in effect on plaque accumulation or gingival health [13]. Chlorhexidine is also useful for patients after orthognathic surgery, especially when inter-maxillary fixation is to be used.

On the other hand, Fluoride mouth rinses significantly reduce the extent of enamel decalcification and gingival inflammation during orthodontic treatment [13.14]. A number of studies evaluated the effect of mechanical aids, as compared with manual tooth brushing, on oral hygiene in orthodontic patients [11.12] and it has been shown that the use of electric tooth-brushes brought a significant improvement in oral hygiene. The orthodontist can follow some suggestions in order to improve plaque removal by the patient. Bonding of molars results in better periodontal health than banding. Whenever possible the use of single arch wires is recommended. The removal of excess composite around brackets, especially at the gingival margin, and avoiding the use of lingual appliances whenever possible are also important ideas in order to keep healthy periodontal tissue during any orthodontic treatment.

3. Periodontal tissue and orthodontics

3.1. Periodontal tissue and orthodontic forces

Tooth movement during orthodontic therapy is the result of placing controlled forces on teeth. Removable appliances place intermittent tipping forces on teeth while fixed appliances can create continuous multidirectional forces to create torquing, intrusive, extrusive, rotational and bodily movement [15.16]. Bone surrounding a tooth subjected to a force responds in the following manner: resorption occurs where there is pressure and new bone forms where there is tension. When pressure is applied to a tooth, there is an initial period of movement for six to eight days as the periodontal ligament (PDL) is compressed. Compression of the PDL results in blood supply being cut off to an area of the PDL and this produces an avascular cell-free zone by a process termed "hyalinization". When hyalinization occurs, the tooth stops moving. Once the hyalinized is removed, tooth movement can occur again [16.17].

3.2. Mechanisms of tissue damage

Unfestooned orthodontic bands are particularly suspects as possibly complicating factors jeopardizing interproximal periodontal support, and at the present time "special periodontally friendly bands" are being designed in research and design laboratories. These challenging effects of band impingement may directly compromise local resistance related to subgingival pathogens in susceptible patients and result in damage to both interproximal gingival tissues and alveolar crestal bone in a manner similar to that produced by faulty crown margins. Periodontal support might also be damaged during tooth intrusion where patients have active periodontitis or gingival infection significant enough to convert to periodontal disease.

The etiology of periodontal problems may not simply rely on exaggerated host immunologic reactions. Mattingly and coworkers [18] and others [19.20.21] reflect the view that long-term fixed appliances can contribute to unfortunate but predictable qualitative alterations in the subgingival bacterial biofilms that become progressively periodontopathic with time.

On a practical level it seems that an absence of bleeding on probing is a better forecasting parameter of health than bleeding on probing is a predictor of progressive disease. In other words, an absence of bleeding on probing, despite the pocket depth can justifiably be used as a test of "healthy gums." On the other hand, while bleeding on probing is certainly an indication of infection of the gingivae, it is one of many risk factors associated with progressive bone loss due to periodontitis. However, the test is not spontaneous bleeding or even bleeding on brushing and flossing. That elicits only superficial disease, one that contributes significantly to caries and marginal decalcification. The best test is "bleeding on probing" elicited by stroking the sulci with a flexible plastic periodontal probe at a comfortable range of force between 10 and 20 g. Those orthodontic patients who present with persistent bleeding on such probing should be notified that they are "at risk" and that prudence dictates a more intensive regimen of periodontal therapy than those who present with little or no bleeding on probing. Since bleeding swollen gingiva is ubiquitous in the orthodontic population, universal caution should be employed and supportive periodontal care recommended routinely as an integral part of orthodontic therapy. Studies have pointed out the importance of a full-mouth examination, six sites per tooth, for a comprehensive description of periodontal status in orthodontic patients [22.23].

3.3. Orthodontic treatment in periodontally susceptible or compromised patients

Under severe control against formation of dental biofilm and elimination or surveillance of periodontal pockets, patients who present susceptible or compromised periodontal status can be submitted to orthodontic treatment [24.25.26]. Moreover, the orthodontic treatment allows that the stable periodontal status is maintained [27.28.29.30]

Although there is no clear correlation between malocclusion and periodontal disease or between the effects of orthodontic treatments on periodontal improvement the literature describes clear interaction between Orthodontics and Periodontics [9].

Probable contributions of orthodontics in the periodontics field are:

1. It allows better oral hygiene by the patient, since it provides well shaped dental arches. Without dental crowding, malocclusion as a periodontal disease facilitator is eliminated;

2.   It allows vertical occlusal impact parallels to the long axes of the teeth. Therefore, the applied muscle force is uniformly distributed all over the dental arch;

3.   It contributes, along with prosthetic rehabilitations, for a normal vertical dimension;

4.   In selected cases, it allows that the adequate dental crown-root relationship is achieved with induced orthodontic extrusion, with no bone loss;

5.   It facilitates that bone vertical defects are corrected or improved with dental uprighting;

6.   It improves the positioning of prosthetic pillars for fixed prostheses and of the next teeth of osteointegrated implants;

7.   It decreases or eliminates effects of bruxism, as pain or muscle spasms, during the orthodontic therapy;

8.   With the current available orthodontic technology and with correct planning and execution, it allows precise, light and efficient orthodontic movements.

Summarizing, when the periodontal inflammatory/infectious process is controlled and the periodontal health is stabilized, the orthodontic treatment is indicated. However, orthodontic movements in periodontal susceptible or compromised patients in active status of inflammation /infection increase significantly the risk of loss of attachment and of bone loss. In extreme cases, they can provoke periodontal collapse and condemnation of the teeth to extraction [9].

4. Combined periodontal/orthodontic treatment

4.1. Periodontal treatment schedule

When planning orthodontic treatment in adults with a history of periodontal disease, it is suggested to allow 2– 6 months from the end of periodontal therapy until bracket placement, for periodontal tissue remodelling, restoration of health and evaluation of patient's compliance. The patient should practise sound oral hygiene and fully understand the potential risks in case of non-compliance [8]. It should be kept in mind that the critical pocket depth for maintaining periodontal health with ordinary oral hygiene is 5–6 mm [31].

During orthodontic treatment, professional cleaning and examination of periodontal tissues should be performed routinely [8]. The specific interval varies for each patient (few weeks to 6 months), and it should be determined considering the analysis of risk factors for periodontal disease and the planned tooth movements. Thorough tooth cleaning and scaling is suggested at short intervals when intrusion and new attachment is attempted 32]. If the patient fails to maintain high level of oral hygiene, orthodontic treatment should be interrupted.

Elective periodontal treatment should be implemented during the final stages of orthodontic treatment or even later, when the final position of hard and soft tissues can be safely determined. The decision is individualized depending on the clinical characteristics of the case and the comprehensive treatment plan [33.34.35].

After the end of active orthodontic treatment and appliance removal, the patient should receive renewed oral hygiene instructions for reducing the risk of recession, because plaque removal and tooth cleaning will be more easily performed. Also, patients should be introduced to a programme of regular follow-up visits to the periodontist and the orthodontist. The timing between follow-up visits is prescribed by the team according to the severity of the patient's pre-treatment condition and the prognosis of the post-treatment condition.

4.2. Treatment phases

4.2.1. Preorthodontic phase

Preorthodontically, the emphasis is on reducing marginal inflammation, augmenting the soft tissue volume in patients with critical mucogingival findings, and improving hygiene conditions through caries therapy and temporary restorations.

The control of periodontal infection by oral hygiene instruction, professional plaque removal and root planing is a fundamental prerequisite for subsequent orthodontic therapy. Many studies have shown that teeth with a reduced but healthy periodontium can be moved without further attachment loss. On the other hand inflammatory periodontal destruction is accelerated by plaque-infected teeth with destroyed connective tissue attachment.

If periodontal regeneration is indicated, a surgical approach is inevitable. Resective bone surgery during flap surgery is contraindicated because orthodontically induced remodeling processes may have a positive influence on osseous topography. Orthodontic treatment can be started 4–6 weeks after the regenerative periodontal therapy; the interaction of progressing regenerative wound healing and orthodontic tissue remodeling may result in additional attachment gain [2].

4.2.2. Orthodontic phase

The orthodontic therapy is determined by two key factors:

- Findings-oriented biomechanics, calculation of active and reactive forces as well as moments as far as possible

- Continuous monitoring of periodontal health. Thorough planning of biomechanics reduces the risk of root resorptions as well as of bone and gingival dehiscences.

A further loss of bone sup-port or attachment induced by uncontrolled force systems should be avoided in all events – especially in patients with periodontally affected teeth.

Maintenance of periodontal health requires meticulous plaque removal in all hygiene-critical areas: bracket periphery, and interproximal and gingival tooth surfaces. If uncontrollable aggravation of the periodontal destruction occurs or if the patient's oral hygiene deteriorates, orthodontic therapy has to be stopped to ensure a reasonable risk/benefit ratio [2].

4.2.3. Postorthodontic phase

The postorthodontic retention phase should last at least six months to permit complete mineralization of osteoid tissues. Only then can the periodontal status be re-evaluated and a decision made on definitive prosthetic measures and the individual retention strategy. For many reasons postorthodontic stability requires semi-permanent or permanent retention:

- to prevent the risk of relapse

- to offset any imbalance of soft tissue/reduced bone support • to eliminate secondary occlusal trauma • to improve masticatory comfort in the presence of increased tooth mobility.

Fixed lingual retainers, passive plates or acrylic foils serve for semi-permanent stabilization, while intracoronal titanium pins are suitable for permanent retention [2].

5. Aspects in periodontic-orthodontic interrelationships

Generally, the main reasons routinely cited to justify the provision of orthodontic treatment are improvement of facial and dental aesthetics and of dental health and function. However, association between malocclusions and periodontal condition is still controversial.

Ngom and co-workers [4] found significant correlations between malocclusions and periodontal condition and suggested that malocclusions are risk markers for periodontal diseases. However, a real inference about a cause/effect relationship between malocclusions and periodontal condition in this study was not possible.

A review of the literature conducted by Van Gastel [5] showed contradictory findings on the impact of malocclusion and orthodontic appliances on periodontal health, since only a few studies reported attachment loss during orthodontic treatment. It has been suggested that this contradiction may be partly due to the selection of materials and differences in the research methods employed. However, our previous studies showed that orthodontic treatment in general does not have any negative effects on the periodontal tissues when a high level of oral hygiene is maintained [6.36].

Actually, between the year 1964 and 2007, sufficient studies had been conducted in terms of orthodontic treatment and possible related periodontal changes. Thus, it sounds plausible to extract evidence-based conclusions from those studies by means of systematic reviews.

In 2008, Bollen [36] conducted two systematic reviews to address the following questions: does a malocclusion affect periodontal health, and does orthodontic treatment affect periodontal health? The first review found a correlation between the presence of a malocclusion and periodontal disease. Subjects with greater malocclusion have more severe periodontal disease. The second review identified an absence of reliable evidence on the effects of orthodontic treatment on periodontal health. The existing low-quality evidence suggests that orthodontic therapy results in small detrimental effects to the periodontium. It has been suggested that the results of both reviews do not warrant recommendation for orthodontic treatment to prevent future periodontal problems, except for specific unusual malocclusions.

In 2010, Van Gastel and co-workers showed in his study [37] that placement of fixed ortho-dontic appliances has an influence both on microbial and clinical periodontal parameters, which were only partly normalized, 3 months following the removal of the appliances.

On the other side, it seems that there still are studies that give the orthodontic treatment positive points regarding periodontal health. Gray and McIntyre [38] conducted a systematic literature review to determine the effectiveness of orthodontic oral health promotion (OHP) upon gingival health, and it has been found that an OHP program for patients undergoing fixed appliance orthodontic treatment produces a short-term reduction (up to 5 months) in plaque and improvement in gingival health.

The results of Gomes and co-workers [39] indicate that use of orthodontics appliances is not necessarily related to a worsening of periodontal conditions. The results of this study reinforce the importance of susceptibility to periodontal disease independent of a well-known retentive plaque factor, i.e. orthodontic appliances and/or bands.

The existing evidence, in general, does not seem to support the claim that orthodontic therapy results in overall improvement in periodontal health.

6. Contribution of orthodontics to periodontal therapy

Orthodontics can serve as an adjunct to periodontal treatment procedures to improve oral health in a number of situations. Pathological tooth migration is one of the few evident signs of periodontitis that affects dentofacial esthetics. This phenomenon is more commonly seen in the anterior dentition due to lack of stable occlusal and sagittal contacts with the opposing teeth [39.40].

Achieving an esthetically acceptable result in such cases may require various orthodontic tooth movements like intrusion, rotation, and uprighting. This can also help control periodontal breakdown and restore good oral function [41].

Tulloch [42] is of the opinion that fixed appliance therapy is more preferable if orthodontic tooth movement is desired in a patient suffering from periodontitis. Fixed appliance allows easy splinting of teeth to achieve stable anchorage. He also highlights the importance of reducing the force magnitude and applying counteracting moments to reduce the stress on periodontal ligament fibres.

Lijian [24] has enlisted the various precautions to be taken when attempting tooth movement in height-reduced periodontium, which includes achieving stable anchorage and long-term periodontal maintenance care.

Deepa [43] reported the use of orthodontic soft aligners in repositioning a periodontally involved tooth. Light and intermittent forces generated by the soft aligner allow regeneration of tissue during tooth movement. Along with periodontal procedures, orthodontically assisted occlusal improvement may be required in treatment of patients with severely attrited lower anterior teeth.

Patient's compliance, motivation, and oral hygiene maintenance will help determine the best time to start adjunctive orthodontic treatment. It is suggested that tooth movement can be undertaken 6 months after completion of active periodontal treatment if there is sufficient evidence of complete resolution of inflammation [44].

Sanders [45] has recommended a three-step comprehensive protocol to be followed before, during, and after adjunctive orthodontic therapy. In patients diagnosed with vertical bony defects, adjunctive orthodontic procedures can help improve the condition. The authors reported improvement in alveolar bone defects, gingival esthetics, and the crown-root ratio in patients with one-or two-wall isolated vertical infrabony defects with a combination of tooth extrusion and periodontal treatment. Orthodontic intrusion has also been shown to improve periodontal condition [46]. However, elimination of pockets was undertaken prior to intrusion in order to prevent apical displacement of plaque [47].

Orthodontic treatment could improve adjacent tooth position before implant placement or tooth replacement. This is especially true for the patient who has been missing teeth for several years and had drifting and tipping of the adjacent dentition

7. Contribution of periodontics to orthodontic therapy

On many occasions, a stable and esthetically acceptable outcome cannot be achieved with orthodontics without adjunctive periodontal procedures. For instance, a high labial frenum attachment is considered to be a causative factor of midline diastema. Frenectomy is recommended in such cases as the fibres are thought to prevent the mesial migration of the central incisors. However, the timing of periodontal intervention has been a topic of much debate [37].

According to Vanarsdall, [49] surgical removal of a maxillary labial frenum should be delayed until after orthodontic treatment unless the tissue prevents space closure or becomes painful and traumatized.

Forced eruption of a labially or palatally impacted tooth is now a common orthodontic treatment procedure. Careful exposure of the impacted tooth while preserving keratinized tissue requires the expertise of a periodontist. Preservation of keratinized tissue is important to prevent loss of attachment. The preferred surgical procedure is primarily an apically or laterally positioned pedicle graft [50].

Retention of orthodontically achieved tooth rotation is a problem that has always plagued the orthodontist. Circumferential supracrestal fiberotomy (CSF) is a procedure that is frequently used to enhance post-treatment stability [50]. Edwards [51] concluded from his long-term prospective study that CSF is more successful in preventing relapse in the maxillary arch. According to him, CSF does not affect the periodontium adversely.

Mucogingival surgeries may be needed during the course of orthodontic treatment to maintain sufficient width of attached gingival [52]. Also, crown lengthening procedures can facilitate easy placement of orthodontic attachments on teeth with short clinical crowns. This procedure can also be used for smile designing [53]. Alveolar ridge augmentation and placements of dental implants [54] are the other adjunctive periodontal treatment procedures undertaken to facilitate achievement of orthodontic treatment goals.

Panwar *et al.* [55] in 2010 presented a case report on combined periodontal and orthodontic treatment of pathologic migration of anterior teeth. Comprehensive orthodontics was initiated with pre-adjusted edgewise appliances using very light force, which resulted in optimal biological response. Since there was trauma from lower anterior teeth, anterior bite plane allowed posterior eruption of teeth, which resulted in the opening of the bite. The periodontal health improved the moment trauma was relieved. Periodontal treatment and the patient's co-operation in oral hygiene were also continued as supportive therapy.

Michael *et al.* in 2009 provided the treatment options for the significant dental midline diastema. After the required prosthetic intervention, periodontal tissues were altered by gingivoplasty and crown lengthening and provided optimal result with favorable esthetic, functional, and biologic consequences [56].

8. Case report

8.1. Case n°1

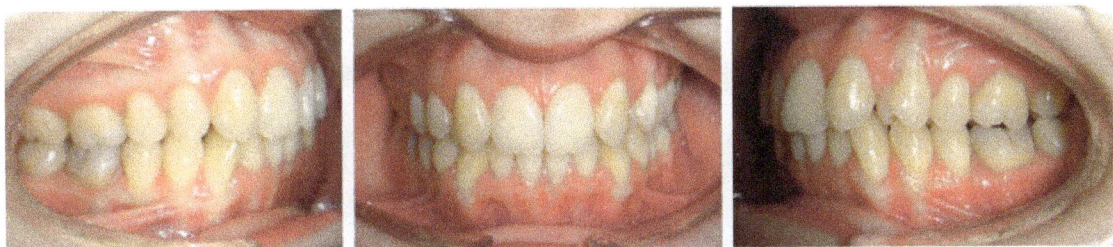

Figure 1. A patient who consults for gingival recession at the 24

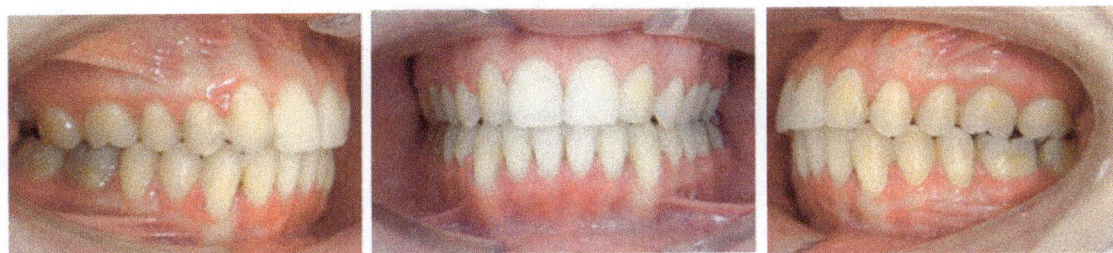

Figure 2. Orthodontic treatment has been used to correct the malocculsion and to correct the rotation of the 24. A gingival grafting was performed to cover the recession

8.2. Case n°2

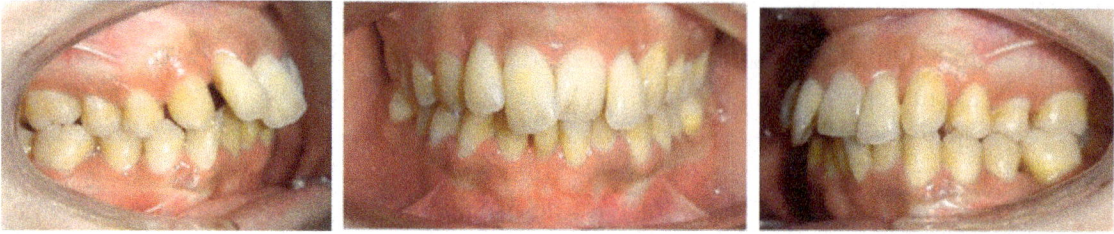

Figure 3. A patient who consults for malpositions and dental extrusions

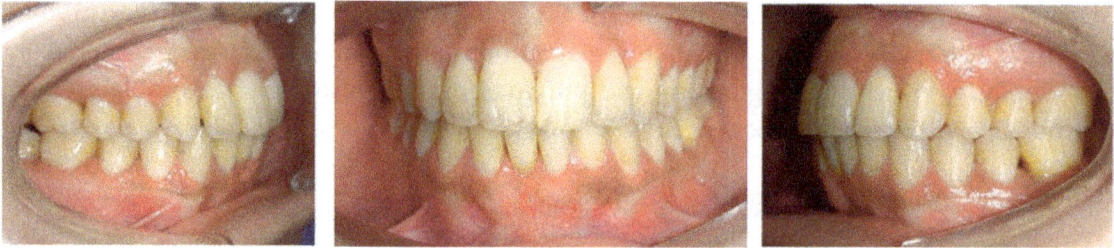

Figure 4. Orthodontic treatment was aimed at correcting dental malposition and regain proper alignment will facilitate the oral hygiene.

8.3. Case n°3

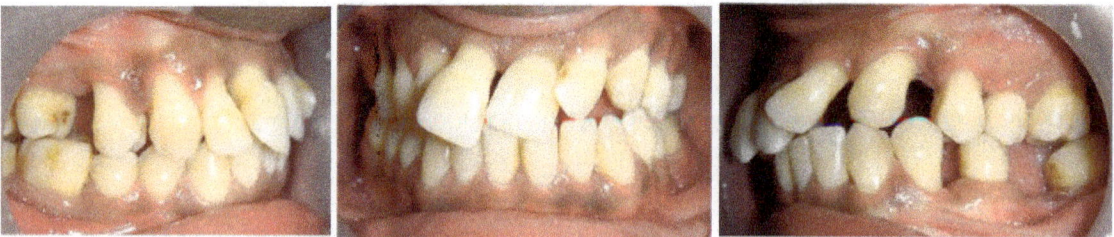

Figure 5. A patient with dental malposition and higher gingival recession secondary to periodontal disease

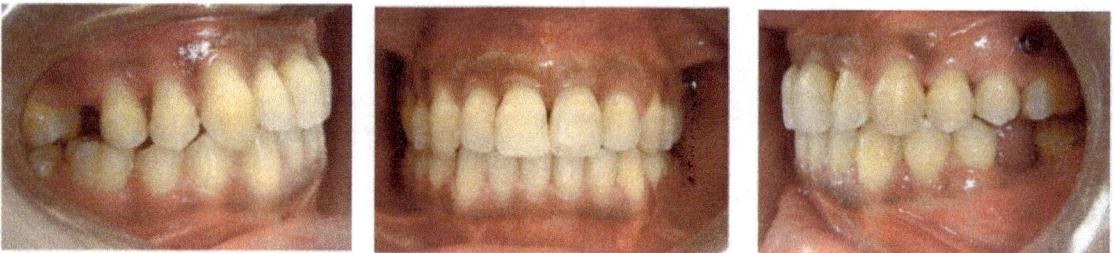

Figure 6. Orthodontic treatment was able to obtain dental and periodontal balance while maintaining good oral hygiene.

8.4. Case n°4

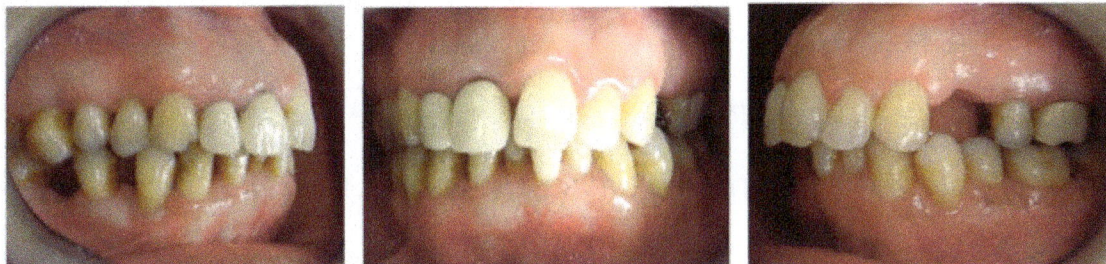

Figure 7. Clinical examination in this patient showed defective prostheses with poor periodontal status.

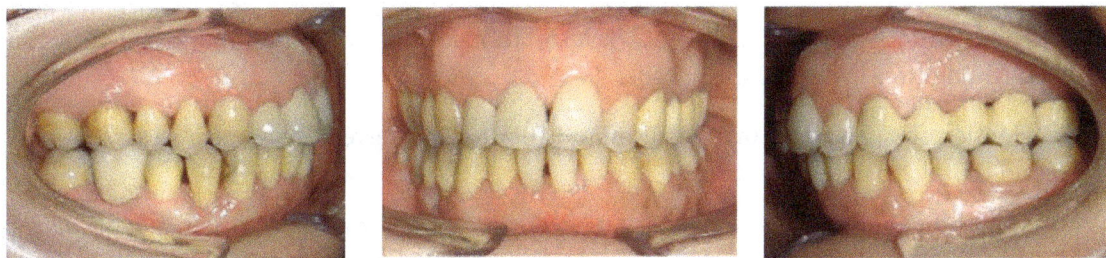

Figure 8. Orthodontic treatment was performed to correct the malocclusion. The patient also received a prosthetic rehabilitation.

9. Conclusion

Harmonious cooperation of the general dentist, the periodontist and the orthodontist offers great possibilities for the treatment of combined orthodontic–periodontal problems. Undoubtedly, application of oral hygiene measures is difficult during orthodontic treatment. Orthodontic treatment along with patient's compliance and absence of periodontal inflammation can provide satisfactory results without causing irreversible damage to periodontal tissues. Furthermore, orthodontic treatment can expand the possibilities of periodontal therapy in certain patients, contributing to better control of microbiota, reducing the potentially hazardous forces applied to teeth and finally improving the overall prognosis. Participation of the periodontist is also essential, either in management of orthodontic–periodontal problems or in specific interventions aiming to prevent orthodontic treatment's relapse.

Author details

Mourad Sebbar[1*], Zouhair Abidine[1], Narjisse Laslami[2] and Zakaria Bentahar[2]

*Address all correspondence to: mouradsebbar@hotmail.com

1 Hospital Moulay Abdellah, Mohammedia, Morocco

2 Department of orthodontics, Faculty of dentistry, Casablanca, Morocco

References

[1] Gkantidis N, Christou P, Topouzelis N. The orthodontic–periodontic interrelationship in integrated treatment challenges: a systematic review. J Oral Rehabilitation 2010;37:377-390.

[2] Diedrich P, Fritz U, Kinzinger G. Interrelationship between Periodontics and Adult Orthodontics Perio 2004,1(3): 143-149.

[3] Dannan A. An update on periodontic-orthodontic interrelationships. J Indian Soc Periodontol 2010,14: 66-71.

[4] Ngom PI, Benoist HM, Thiam F, Diagne F, Diallo PD. Influence of orthodontic anomalies on periodontal condition. Odontostomatol Trop 2007;301:9-16.

[5] Van Gastel J, Quirynen M, Teughels W, Carels C. The relationships between malocclusion, fixed orthodontic appliances and periodontal disease: A review of the literature. Aust Orthod J 2007;23:121-9.

[6] Dannan A, Darwish MA, Sawan MN. Effect of orthodontic tooth movements on the periodontal tissues. Damascus Univ Journal for Health Sciences [Master Thesis] 2005;21:306-7.

[7] Dannan A, Darwish MA, Sawan MN. How do the periodontal tissues react during the orthodontic alignment and leveling phase? Virtual J Orthod 2008;8:1-7.

[8] Sanders NL. Evidence-based care in orthodontics and periodontics: a review of the literature. J Am Dent Assoc. 1999;130(4):521-7.

[9] Del Santo M. Periodontium and Orthodontic Implications: Clinical Applications. Int J Stomatol Res 2012, 1(3): 17-23.

[10] Jackson CL. Comparison between electric toothbrushing and manual toothbrushing, with and without oral irrigation, for oral hygiene of orthodontic patients. Am J Orthod Dentofacial Orthop. 1991;99(1):15-20.

[11] Wilcoxon DB, Ackerman RJ, Jr., Killoy WJ, Love JW, Sakumura JS, Tira DE. The effectiveness of a counterrotational-action power toothbrush on plaque control in orthodontic patients. Am J Orthod Dentofacial Orthop. 1991;99(1):7-14.

[12] Brightman LJ, Terezhalmy GT, Greenwell H, Jacobs M, Enlow DH. The effects of a 0.12% chlorhexidine gluconate mouthrinse on orthodontic patients aged 11 through 17 with established gingivitis. Am J Orthod Dentofacial Orthop. 1991;100(4):324-9.

[13] Pontier JP, Pine C, Jackson DL, DiDonato AK, Close J, Moore PA. Efficacy of a pre-brushing rinse for orthodontic patients. Clin Prev Dent. 1990;12(3):12-7.

[14] Denes J, Gabris K. Results of a 3-year oral hygiene programme, including amine fluoride products, in patients treated with fixed orthodontic appliances. Eur J Orthod. 1991;13(2):129-33.

[15] Lindhe J. Textbook of clinical periodontology. 2nd ed. Copenhagen: Munksgaard; 1989.

[16] Proffit WR, Fields HW. Contemporary orthodontics. 2nd ed. St Louis: CV Mosby; 1993.

[17] Reitan K. Biomechanical principles and reactions. In: Graber X, Swain BF, editors. Current orthodontic concepts and techniques. St Louis: CV Mosby; 1985. p. 101-92.

[18] Mattingly JA, Sauer GJ, Yancey JM, Arnold RR. Enhancement of 27. streptococcus mutans colonization by direct bonded orthodontic appliances. J Dent Res 1983;62:1209-11.

[19] Paolantonio M, Festa F, di Placido G, D'Attilio M, Catamo28. G, Piccolomini R. Site-specific subgingival colonization by actinobacillus actinomycetemcomitans in orthodontic patients. Am J Orthod Dentofacial Orthop 1999;115:423-8.

[20] Sallum A, et al. Clinical and microbiologic changes after removal of orthodontic appliances. Am J Orthod Dentofacial Orthop 2004;126:363-6.

[21] Perinetti G, Paolantonio M, Serra E, D'Archivio D, D'Ercole S, Festa F, et al. Longitudinal monitoring of subgingival colonization by actinobacillus actinomycetemcomitans, and crevicular alkaline phosphatise and aspartate aminotransferase activities around orthodontically treated teeth. J Clin Periodontol 2004;31:60-7.

[22] Lijian L. Periodontic-orthodontic interactions—rationale, sequence and clinical implications. Hong Kong Dent J 2007;4:60-4.

[23] Lang NP, Loe H. The relationship between the width of keratinized gingiva and gingival health. J Periodontol 1972;43:623-7.

[24] Elliasson LA, Hugoson A, Kurol J, Siwe H. The effects of orthodontic treatment on periodontal tissues in patients with reduced periodontal support. Eur J Orthod 1982;4:1-9.

[25]   Boyd RL, Leggot PJ, Quinn RS, Eakle WS, Chambers DW. Periodontal implications of orthodontic treatment in adults with reduced or normal periodontal tissues versus those of adolescents. Am J Orthod Dentofac Orthop 1989;96:191-8.

[26]   Ong M A Wang HL. Periodontic and orthodontic treatment in adults. Am J Orthod Dentofac Orthop 2002;122:420-8.

[27]   Brown S The effect of orthodontic therapy on certain types of periodontal defects (I). Clinical findings. J Periodontol 1973;44:742-56.

[28]   Ingber JS. Forced eruption. Part I. A method of treating isolated one and two wall infrabony osseous defects – rationale and case report. J Periodontol 1974;45:199-206.

[29]   Ingber JS. Forced eruption. Part II. A method of treating nonrestorable teeth – periodontal and restorative considerations. J Periodontol 1976;47:203-16.

[30]   Kraal JH, Digiancinto JJ, Dail RA. Lemmerman K, Peden JW. Periodontal conditions in patients after molar uprighting. J Prosth Dent 1980;43:156-62.

[31]   Socransky SS, Haffajee AD. The nature of periodontal diseases. Ann Periodontol. 1997;2:3–10.

[32]   Melsen B, Agerbaek N, Markenstam G. Intrusion of incisors in adult patients with marginal bone loss. Am J Orthod Dentofacial Orthop. 1989;96:232–241.

[33]   Spear FM, Kokich VG, Mathews DP. Interdisciplinary man-agement of anterior dental esthetics. J Am Dent Assoc 2006;137:160–169.

[34]   Konikoff BM, Johnson DC, Schenkein HA, Kwatra N, Waldrop TC. Clinical crown length of the maxillary anterior teeth preorthodontics and postorthodontics. J Periodontol. 2007;78:645–653.

[35]   Theytaz GA, Kiliaridis S. Gingival and dentofacial changes in adolescents and adults 2 to 10 years after orthodontic treatment. J Clin Periodontol. 2008;35:825–830.

[36]   Bollen AM. Effects of malocclusions and orthodontics on periodontal health: Evidence from a systematic review. J Dent Educ 2008;72:912-8.

[37]   Van Gastel J, Quirynen M, Teughels W, Coucke W, Carels C. Longitudinal changes in microbiology and clinical periodontal parameters after removal of fixed orthodontic appliances. Eur J Orthod 2011;33:15-21.

[38]   Gray D, McIntyre G. Does oral health promotion influence the oral hygiene and gingival health of patients undergoing fixed appliance orthodontic treatment? A systematic literature review. J Orthod 2008;35:262-9.

[39]   Gomes SC, Varela CC, da Veiga SL, Rösing CK, Oppermann RV. Periodontal conditions in subjects following orthodontic therapy. A preliminary study. Eur J Orthod. 2007;29(5):477-81.

[40]   Vinod K, Reddy YG, Reddy VP, Nandan H, Sharma M. Orthodontic-periodontics interdisciplinary approach. J Indian Soc Periodontol. 2012;16(1):11-5.

[41] Zachrisson BU. Orthodontics and periodontics. In: Lindhe J, Karring T, Lang NP, editors. Clinical periodontology and implant dentistry. 4th ed. Oxford: Blackwell Munksgaard; 2003:744-80.

[42] Tulloch JF. Adjunctive treatment for adults. In: Proffit WR, Fields J r HW, editors. Contemporary orthodontics. 3rd ed. St. Louis: Mosby; 2000:616-43.

[43] Deepa D, Mehta DS, Puri VK, Shetty S. Combined periodontic-orthodontic-endodontic interdisciplinary approach in the treatment of periodontally compromised tooth. J Indian Soc Periodontol 2010;14:139-43.

[44] Padmanabhan S, Reddy VL. Inter-disciplinary management of a patient with severely attrited teeth. J Indian Soc Periodontol 2010;14:190-4.

[45] Sanders NL. Evidence-based care in orthodontics and periodontics: A review of the literature. J Am Dent Assoc 1999;130:521-7.

[46] Lino S, Taira K, Machigashira M, Miyawaki S. Isolated vertical infrabony defects treated by orthodontic tooth extrusion. Angle Orthod 2008;78:728-36.

[47] Sam K, Rabie AB, King NM. Orthodontic intrusion of periodontally involved teeth. J Clin Orthod 2001;35:325-30.

[48] Melsen B. Tissue reaction following application of extrusive and intrusive forces to teeth in adult monkeys. Am J Orthod 1986;89:469-75.

[49] Vanarsdall RE. Periodontal/orthodontic interrelationships. In: Graber TM, Vanarsdall RE, editors. Orthodontics-current principles and technique. 3rd ed. St. Louis: Mosby; 2000:801-38.

[50] Vanarsdall RL, Corn H. Soft-tissue management of labially positioned unerupted teeth. Am J Orthod 1977;72:53-64.

[51] Edwards JG. A surgical procedure to eliminate rotational relapse. Am J Orthod 1970;57:35-46.

[52] Edwards JG. A long-term prospective evaluation of the circumferential supracrestal-fiberotomy in alleviating orthodontic relapse. Am J Orthod Dentofacial Orthop 1988;93:380-7.

[53] Kokich VG. Esthetics: The orthodontic-periodontic restorative connection. Semin Orthod 1996;2:21-30.

[54] Huang LH, Shotwell JL, Wang HL. Dental implants for orthodonticanchorage. Am J Orthod Dentofacial Orthop 2005;127:713-22.

[55] Panwar M, Jayan B. Combined periodontal and orthodontic treatment of pathologic migration of anterior teeth. MJAFI 2010;66:67-9.

[56] Michael R. Treatment options for the significant dental midline diastema inside dentistry 2009. http:/www.dentalaegis.com/id/2009/05/clinical-treatment-options-treatment-optionsfor-the-significant-dental-midline-diastema.

4

Clinical Consideration and Management of Impacted Maxillary Canine Teeth

Belma Işık Aslan and Neslihan Üçüncü

1. Introduction

Impaction is a retardation or halt in the normal process of tooth. There are various terminology in literature to define impaction including delayed eruption, primary retention, submerged teeth, impacted teeth ets. A canine is considered as being impacted if it is interrupted after complete root development or the contralateral tooth is erupted for at least 6 months with complete root formation [1].

Impaction of maxillary canines is a frequently encountered clinical problem. The cause of canine impaction can be the result of localized, systemic or genetic factor(s). There are a number of possible sequelae to canine impactions. The diagnosis and localization of the impacted canines is the most important step in the management of impacted canines based on clinical and radiographic examinations. Treatment of impacted maxillary canines usually requires an interdisciplinary approach. Treatment options include no treatment, interseptive approach, extraction, autotransplantation and surgical exposure and orthodontic alignment of the impacted canine. The most desirable treatment approach is early diagnosis and interception of potential impaction. However, in the absence of prevention, surgical exposure and orthodontic alignment should be considered. Surgical treatment techniques and orthodontic considerations depend on the location of the impacted canine in the dental arch.

2. Incidance of impacted canines

Maxillary canines are the second-most frequently impacted teeth after the third molars [2] with prevalence from 0.8-5.2 % depending on the population examined [3,4]. The incidence of maxillary canine impaction is about 20 times more than mandibular canine impaction [5].

Approximately one third of impacted maxillary canines are positioned labially or within the alveolus, and two thirds are located palatally [6]. In another study [7], Ericson and Kurol reported that, 50% of the 156 ectopically positioned canines were in a palatal or distopalatal position, 39% in a buccal or distobuccal position, and 11% apical to the adjacent incisor or between the roots of the central and lateral incisors. Maxillary canine impactions occur twice as often in females than in males [8] and only 8% of canine impactions are bilateral [9].

3. Developmental considerations

Maxillary canines develop lateral to the priform fossa and have a longer and difficult path of eruption than any other tooth through they reach their final position in occlusion. Coulter and Richardson [10] stated that in three planes of space, maxillary canines travel almost 22 mm from their position at the age of 5 years to their position at 15 years. At the age of 3 maxillary canine is high in the maxilla, with its crown directed mesially and lingually. At the age of 8 it angulates medially with its crown lying distal and slightly buccal to the lateral incisor [11]. Also at this stage the canine normally migrates buccally from a position lingual to the root apex of its deciduous precursor, however, if it cannot make this transition from the palatal to the buccal side, it remains palatally impacted [12]. Maxillary canines follow a mesial path until it reaches the distal aspect of the lateral incisor root and gradually uprights to a more vertical position by moving towards the occlusal plane guided by the lateral incisor root. However, maxillary canines often erupt into the oral cavity with a marked mesial inclination [13]. If the lateral incisors are congenitally missing, the canine may erupt in a mesial direction until it comes into contact with the distal aspect of the central incisor root and erupts into the lateral incisor space [14]. Consequently, the roots of the lateral incisors play an important role in the guidance of upper permanent canines [15].

Table 1 shows the calcification and eruption timing of the maxillary canines according to Brand and Isselhard [16].

Calcification begins	4 months
Enamel complete	6-7 years
Eruption	11-12 years
Root completed	13-15 years

Table 1. Calcification and eruption timing of the maxillary canines

The mean eruption age for the maxillary canine is approximately 1 year earlier in females (10.98 years) than in males (11.69 years) [17]. Hurme [17] suggested that if maxillary canine has not appeared by the age of 13.1 in males or by 12.3 in females, the eruption may be considered late.

4. Etiology of impacted canines

Eruption is a tightly coordinated process, regulated by a series of signaling effects between the dental follicle and the osteoblast and osteoclast cells found in the alveolar bone [18]. A wide variety of localized, systemic and genetic reasons may cause disruption in eruption process, ranging from delayed eruption to a complete failure of eruption [19]. Systemic reasons include endocrine deficiencies, febrile diseases, and irradiation. There is not only one etiology to explain the occurrence of a majority of impactions or either the localization of impaction occuring labially or palatally [20]. Environmental factors may cause impaction during the long, tortuous eruption path of a canine. The primary causes of impacted canines are localized conditions and result of one or a combination of following factors [21]:

1.   tooth size, arch length discrepancies,

2.   prolonged retention or early loss of the deciduous canine,

3.   apical periodontitis of deciduous teeth [22],

4.   abnormal position of the tooth bud,

5.   presence of an alveolar cleft,

6.   ankylosis,

7.   premature root closure [23],

8.   cystic or neoplastic formation,

9.   dilesaration of the root,

10. disturbances in tooth eruption sequence,

11. mucosal barriers-scar tissue: trauma/surgery [24],

12. gingival fibromatosis/ gingival hyperplasia [25],

13. supernumerary teeth [26],

14. iatrogenic,

15. idiopathic including primary failure of eruption [27].

If no physical barrier can be identified, the cessation of eruption of a normally placed and developed tooth germ before emergence is described as primary retention [28]. Generally genetic etiology is related with primary retention [29]. If the teeth becomes impacted due to an obstruction of the eruption pathway such as crowded dental arch, it is defined as secondary retention [28].

The etiology of impacted teeth may depend upon the location of impacted tooth. The exact etiology of palatally displaced maxillary canines is unknown yet hypothesized to be both multifactorial and genetic in origin [30]. Where as buccal canine impaction is result of ectopic migration of the canine crown over the root of the lateral incisor due to crowding or shifting of the maxillary dental midline, causing insufficient space for the canine to erupt [31].

Two main theories have been associated with the occurrence of palatally impacted maxillary canines: the "guidance theory" and the "genetic theory" [2]. According to the guidance theory, the presence of the lateral incisor root with right length and formed at the right time are important variables needed to guide the mesially erupting canine in a more favorable distal and incisal direction. If excessive space exists due to malformed or absent lateral incisor the canine would cross back from the buccal to the palatal side behind the buds of the other teeth [3]. In the clinical observation of Jacoby [32], he stated that 85% of the 40 palatally impacted canines had sufficient space for eruption in the dental arch. He claimed that labially impacted maxillary canine could only be due to arch length deficiency where as palatal impaction due to excessive space in the canine area. In accordance, Al-Nimri and Gharaibeh [33] stated that the presence of an excess palatal width and anomalous lateral incisor may contribute to the etiology of palatal canine impaction. They have also found that palatal canine impaction occurred most frequently in subjects with a Class II division 2 malocclusion. Conversely, McConnell [34] found transverse maxillary deficiency in palatally impacted canine cases. On the other hand, Langberg and Peck [35] observed no statistically significant difference in the anterior and posterior maxillary arch widths between subjects with palatally displaced canines and a comparison sample.

The genetic theory assigns genetic factors as the primary origin of the eruption anomaly of maxillary permanent canines. Palatally impacted canines, such as familial and bilateral occurrence, sex differences, are genetically associated with dental anomalies such as ectopic eruption of first molars, infraocclusion of primary molars, aplasia of premolars and one third molar [36]. Sacerdoti and Baccetti [38] showed that unilateral palatal canine displacement was associated with missing upper lateral incisors where as bilateral canine displacement with agenesis of third molars, indicating the genetic etiology of palatal canine displacement. Peck et al., [37] also found a positive correlation between palatally displaced canines and third molar agenesis.

5. Sequelae of canine impaction

Careful observation of the development and eruption of canines during periodic dental examination of the growing child is essential to prevent potential complications. Shafer et al. [39] suggested the following sequelae for canine impaction:

1. labial or lingual malpositioning of the impacted tooth,

2. migration of the neighboring teeth and loss of arch length,

3. internal resorption,

4. dentigerous cyst formation,

5. external root resorption of the impacted tooth, as well as the neighboring teeth,

6.   infection particularly with partial eruption, and

7.   referred pain and combinations of the above sequelae.

6. Diagnosis of impacted canines

The diagnosis and localization of the impacted canines is the most important step in the management of impacted canines based on clinical and radiographic examinations.

6.1. Clinical evaluation

In clinical evaluation firstly patient's age and dentition should be examined to detemine whether there is a delayed eruption or not. Secondly, the presence or absence of a factor such as certain diseases that may cause tooth structure, size, shape, and color defects adversely affecting tooth development should be searched [40]. Subsequently the amount of space in the arch for the unerupted canine, the morphology and position of the adjacent teeth, the contours of the bone, the mobility of teeth should be considered through clinical evaluation [41].

Indicative clinical signs of canine impaction may be listed as following: [20]

1.   delayed eruption of the permanent canine or prolonged retention of the deciduous canine beyond 14 to 15 years of age,

2.   the presence of an asymmetry in the canine bulge or absence of a normal labial canine bulge observed during alveolar palpation,

3.   presence of a palatal bulge, and

4.   distal tipping, or migration of the lateral incisor

During normal eruption of the maxillary canine, usually a labial bulge is noted on the mucosa superior to the maxillary primary canine. When such a bulge is not visible, an intraoral palpation is required to provide a clear localization of the permanent canine. Also mobility of all present teeth should be assessed during palpation. Mobile deciduous canines may indicate normal resorption of the roots by the permanent canines where as mobility of the permanent lateral incisor may be the potential result of root resorption by the impacted canine [20].

According to Ericson and Kurol [42] the absence of the "canine bulge" at earlier ages should not be considered as indicative of canine impaction. In their evaluation of 505 schoolchildren between 8 and 12 years of age, they found that at 10 years, 29% of the children had nonpalpable canines, but only 5% at 11 years of age, whereas at later ages only 3% had nonpalpable canines. They found that many of the children under 10 years of age whose canines initially were determined by palpation to be potentially abnormal, actually later developed and erupted normally. Thus they found radiographic examination impractical and unnecessary for children under 10 years of age [43].

In contrast, examination of intrabony movement of the canines between the dental age of 8 to 10 years was advised by Williams [44]. If permanent canine bulges are not palpable, he offered to examine lateral and frontal radiographs specifically for Class I malocclusions, even with minimal arch length loss. He suggested removing the deciduous canine when a position apparently lingual to the anterior teeth on the lateral radiograph and a medial tilt of the long axis of the canine in relation to the lateral wall of the nasal cavity on the frontal radiograph are observed.

6.2. Radiographic verification

The accurate location of impacted canines and determining their relationship to adjacent incisors and anatomical structures is the part of the diagnostic process and is essential for successful treatment. This required information can be partially obtained from conventional two-dimensional radiographs as the first step which includes periapical radiographs, occlusal films, panoramic views, and lateral cephalograms [45].

In most cases analysis should begin with routine periapical films. A single periapical film would relate the canine with the neighboring teeth both mesiodistally and superoinferiorly. In order to estimate the buccolingual position of the canine, a second periapical film is obtained by using [46]: (1) Tube-shift technique or Clark's rule, (2) buccal-object rule.

In tube-shift technique two adjacent periapical radiographs of the impacted tooth are taken at slightly different horizontal angles. The object that moves in the same direction as the cone, is palatally impacted. If the impacted canine is located buccally, the crown of the tooth moves in the opposite direction as the x-ray beam. Consequently the object closest to the film will move in the same direction as the tube head.

In the buccal-object rule two periapical films are taken of the same area, with approximately 20° vertical angulation of the cone changed when the second film is taken. The buccal object will move in opposite direction to the source of radiation.

Occlusal films also aid to detect the buccolingual position of the impacted canine in conjunction with the periapical films especially when treating an uncooperative child, a child with very small oral aperture. However, alone, this type of radiograph provides no information relative to the vertical position of the impacted tooth [47].

Frontal and lateral cephalograms can sometimes be useful in determining the position of the impacted canine, particularly its relationship to other facial structures, such as the maxillary sinus and the floor of the nose.

Panoramic radiography has also been utilized as a diagnostic tool for determination of unerupted canine positions [48]. Radiographic variables on panoramic x-rays: α-angle (angle measured between the long axis of the impacted canine and the midline), d-distance (distance between the canine cusp tip and the occlusal plane), and s-sector where the cusp of the impacted canine is located (sector 1, between the midline and the axis of the central incisor; sector 2, between the axes of the central incisor and the lateral incisor; or sector 3, between the axes of the lateral incisor and the first premolar) have been shown to be predictive factors for prediction of eventual impaction, the durations of orthodontic traction and comprehensive orthodontic treatment to reposition the impacted tooth. However these features are not valid predictors of the final periodontal status of orthodontically-repositioned impacted canines [49]. The more severely displaced the canine with regard to the adjacent maxillary incisors, the longer the orthodontic treatment.

Medical computerized tomography (CT) was an improvement which overcomes the limitations of conventional two-dimensional (2D) imaging however, radiation exposure of CT scans limits its clinical utility [50]. The advent of 3D cone beam computed tomography (CBCT) has reduced the radiation dose, making it an advantageous tool in dentistry [51]. CBCT images have been proven to be useful for the accurate diagnosis of the impacted canines, treatment planning and the identification of associated complications, such as root resorption in adjacent incisors. In addition it was found that CBCT reduces the treatment duration and increases the success of treatment in difficult cases to a similar level of simpler cases [52]. Small volume CBCT may be indicated as a supplement to a routine panoramic X-ray in the following cases if: [53]

- canine inclination in the panoramic X-ray exceeds 30°

- root resorption of adjacent teeth is suspected

- the canine apex is not clearly discernible in the panoramic X-ray, implying dilaceration of the canine root.

6.3. Root resorption and radiographic evaluation

The ability to evaluate the condition of the lateral incisor root is of great importance to the clinician because 80% of the teeth resorbed by the ectopically erupting canines were found to be lateral incisors [21]. Lateral incisor image could only be evaluated in 37% of the cases with the use of periapical films [47]. However CBCT provides more detailed information about the location and extent of the resorbed roots and may notably alter the prevalence of root resorption [54].

Ericson and Kurol [7] found the incidance of lateral resorption as 38%, in a study of 156 ectopically impacted maxillary canines with using CT. In a more recent study, Oberoi and Knueppel [55] determined no root resorption in 40.4%, slight root resorption in 35.7%, moderate resorption in 14.2% and severe root resorption in 4% of the adjacent lateral incisor evaluated by CBCT.

7. Treatment planning considerations

Maxillary canines play an important role in creating good facial and smile esthetics, since they are positioned at the corners of the dental arch, forming the canine eminence for support of the alar base and the upper lip. Moreover, when the maxillary canines are properly aligned and have good shape and size, pleasing anterior dental proportions and correct smile lines are achieved. Functionally, they support the dentition, contributing to disarticulation during lateral movements in certain persons [56]. Treatment of impacted maxillary canines usually requires an interdisciplinary approach involving oral surgical, restorative, periodontic as well as orthodontic components. Prudent treatment planning is necessary to achieve the various treatment goals [21].

The patient with an impacted maxillary canine initially must undergo a comprehensive clinical and radiographic evalution of the malocclusion to localize the impacted canine and decide on its prognosis for alignment. Patient's cooperation, age, general oral health, skeletal variation and presence of spacing or crowding in the arch are important agents affecting prognosis [57]. Any root resorption of the adjacent teeth should also be considered. Orthoontist should also be aware of the normal development and eruption pattern in order to conduct interceptive treatment if appropriate, which provides cost benefit than other more invasive prosedures. Patient and parent counselling on the treatment options and informed constent is essential to avoid any medicolegal problems [58].

8. Treatment options

The clinician should consider the various treatment options available for the patient, including: [21]

1. No treatment

2. Interseptive treatment

3. Extraction of the impacted canine

4. Autotransplantation of the canine

5. Surgical exposure and orthodontic alignment

1.   No treatment

No active treatment could be recommended when: [59]

• the patient does not request treatment

• there is no sign of resorption of adjacent teeth or other pathology

• there is a severely displaced canine with no evidence of pathology, if it is remote from the dentition ideally there is a good contact between lateral incisor and first premolar or good esthetics/prognosis for deciduous canine

In this instance, the unerupted canine should be periodically monitored with respect to cystic degeneration, root resorption and the other possible complications. The optimal time interval between radiographs is not known to reduce the radiation dosage. In most cases, long-term prognosis of retained deciduous canine is poor, regardless of its root length and crown shape since the root of retained deciduous canine will eventually resorb and it will have to be extracted [21].

2.   Interseptive treatment

Early diagnosis and intervention is very important for it could save the time, expense, and more complex treatment in the permanent dentition. If early signs of ectopic eruption of the canines is determined, the clinician should made an attempt to prevent their impaction and its potential sequalae. Frequently, primary canines are extracted as an interceptive measure to facilite the permanent canine eruption or at least provide changes to a more favorable position [12]. The extraction of the primary canine is recommended when:

- the patient is aged 10-13 years.

- the maxillary canine is not palpable in its normal position and radiographic examination exhibites palatal canine ectopia. If the permanent canine is located in a more medial position or the patient is older than the ideal age group, extraction of the primary canine may provide less favourable results [60].

Clinical re-evaluation and follow-up radiographs should normally be taken at 6-month intervals. If there is no improvement in canine position within 12 months on panaromic films after the extraction of primary canines, an alternative treatment is indicated [61].

The severity of the angulation of the impacted canine is an important factor in the prognosis. The more inclined the tooth is, the less is the probability that it will spontaneously erupt [61]. Power and Short [62] predicted the chances of canine impaction based on orthopantomographs between the years of 10-13 and claimed that eruption chance of the impacted tooth will decrease even after deciduous extraction is performed if the permanent canine is angled more than 31° to the midline.

Ericson and Kurol [61] stated that the removal of the deciduous canine before 11 years of age will normalize the position of the ectopically erupting permanent canines up to 91% if the permanent canine crown is distal to the midline of the lateral incisor. However the success rate decreases to 64% when the canine crown overlaps medially to the long axis midline of the lateral incisor.

Williams [44] suggested the extraction of the maxillary deciduous canine as early as 8 or 9 years of age to enhance the eruption and self-correction of a labial or intra-alveolar maxillary canine impaction in Class I uncrowded cases.

Extraction of deciduous canines in conjunction with the use of cervical pull headgear, and rapid maxillary expansion have been reported to be effective procedures in the interceptive treatment of maxillary canine impaction [2]. Baccetti et al. [63] found that 65 percent of palatally displaced cases that underwent the removal of the deciduous canine resulted in successful eruption of permanent canines without any other treatment. The prevalence rate could be improved significantly up to 88 percent by preventing mesial migration of the upper posterior teeth after extraction of the deciduous canine, such as with the use of cervical-pull headgear [63]. Also Olive [64] stated that opening space for the canine crown with routine orthodontic mechanics might allow for spontaneous eruption of an impacted canine. However early correction of the flared and distally tipped lateral incisors is not recommended in order not to cause impaction of the canines or the resorption of lateral incisor roots [65].

Another randomized clinical trial performed by Bagetti et al. [66] reported that TPA and deciduous canine extraction alone was as effective as rapid maxillary expansion followed by a TPA coupled with the extraction of deciduous canines, as an interceptive treatment option for patients from 9 years 5 months to 13 years of age with palatally displaced canines. The use of these protocols in late mixed dentition subjects increased the eruption rate significantly more than only extraction and untreated groups.

3.   Extraction of impacted canines

The surgical removal of impacted canines although seldom considered might be a viable option in the following situations: [29]

- patient declines active treatment and/or is happy with apperance.

- there is evidence of early resorption of adjacent teeth.

- the patient is too old for interseption.

- there is a good contact for lateral incisor and first premolar or the patient is willing to undergo orthodontic treatment to substitute first premolar for the canine

- if the impacted canine is ankylosed and cannot be transplanted

- if the root of impacted canine is severely dilacerated

- if the impaction is severe and the degree of malocclusion is too great for surgical repositioning/transplantation.

Especially extraction of the labially erupting and crowded canine is contraindicated. Such an extraction might temporarily improve the aesthetics however may complicate and compromise the orthodontic treatment results.

If removal of the impacted canine is required, the orthodontist should decide whether to replace the premolar into the canine position or restore the missing canine space with a prosthesis or an implant. If the canine space is going to be closed orthodontically, the posterior segment has to be protracted. Before the extraction decision is made, factors such as lingual cusp interferences, tooth size discrepancy, and the difficulties encountered when employing unilateral mechanics should also be considered [21].

When an extraction is performed, it often leaves a critical alveolar defect of difficult management. Puricelli et al. [67] recommended maxillary partial osteotomy as an efficient resolution for the correction of bone defects within the dental arches which is performed by mobilizing an alveolar bone segment. They have indicated this technique within the concept of individual and multiple sustenance of integrity in occlusion and of the dental arches, especially in young patients, where the indication for fixed prosthetics or osseointegrated implants might be precocious. They stated that this technique offers a superior time efficient solution for the loss of the maxillary canines compared to the osseointegrated implant rehabilitation or orthodontic space closure.

Surgical extraction of impacted canines and their substitution by first premolars eliminates all the risks and uncertainty related to orthodontic extrusion of an impacted canine. Good functional and esthetic results can be achieved, if an accurate and detailed anterior tooth position is managed during orthodontic finishing [68]. Smile esthetics of maxillary premolar substitution can be improved by intruding the first premolars to a higher gingival margin with respect to the maxillary lateral incisors and restoring the premolars with composite resin buildups or porcelain veneers to produce natural canines [69]. Otherwise slightly extrusion of the maxillary first premolars is also acceptable if premolar crowns are long, with prominent buccal cusps. Also, slight negative crown torque and a mesiopalatal rotation is recommended to resemble a natural canine as possible [68]. Additionally it is reported that there is no scientific evidence that one occlusal scheme is better than the other. Hence canine guidance can well be constructed by premolar guidance or a group function, by slightly extruding the maxillary first premolar [70].

4.   Autotransplantation of the canine

Autotransplantation could be performed as a treatment option when: [59]

* interceptive treatment is inconvenient or has failed,

* the degree of malocclusion is too severe to achieve orthodontic alignment,(crown tip mesial to the mid-line of the lateral incisor or mesial angulation greater than 55° [47],

* adequate space is available for the canine

* the prognosis is good for the tooth to be transplanted and it can be removed atraumatically.

* patient refuses a conventional orthodontic therapy

* failure of orthodontic alignment due to immobility

Successful prognosis of transplanted teeth depends on the following factors: the condition of the remaining periodontal ligament attached to the extracted donor tooth [72], the adaptation of the donor tooth to the socket [73], the duration and the method of splinting after transplantation [74], and the timing of endodontic treatment of the transplanted teeth [75].

Recent studies of autotransplantation of canines have reported success rates of 38–58% over more than 10 years [76, 77]. In another recent study, Huth et al. [71] found that the success rate of autotransplanted teeth was 74%, along with a high patient satisfaction [37]. They recommended autotransplantation especially in adolescent patients in whom alternative treatments, such as dental implants, are not yet indicated since autotransplanted teeth increase or at least maintain the bone level and facilitate a later dental implant supply.

The most relevant complications in autotransplantation of teeth that affect the success rate are inflammatory or replacement resorption [78]. Periodontal healing is responsible for root resorption after autotransplantation. At a later stage of development the root is fully formed and the chances of pulpal and periodontal healing is reduced [79, 80]. The optimal developmental stage for autotransplantation is when the root is 50-75 percent is formed [81].

In some clinical studies it was suggested that the preapplication of mechanical stimuli to the donor teeth might stimulate the periodontal ligament, prevent ankylosis, reduce the damage to the periodontal ligament, and prevent root resorption after replantation [82,83]. Recently,

Ru and Bai [84] reported a maxillary canine autotransplantation case where the extraction site of deciduous canine was preserved with a titanium prosthesis and a bioresorbable membrane to prevent root resorption and anyklosis.

The prognosis of ectopic canine autotransplantation in adults is poor. In the research of Schatz and Joho [85] on 20 transplanted maxillary canines, they determined that pulp vitality remained in 80% of the patients aged 13 to 20 years group however all impacted canines required root canal therapy in the 20-to 48-year age-group.

Endodontic treatment of autotransplanted teeth with closed apices is considered as mandatory analog of traumatically avulsed teeth with closed apices [86]. If the toot has a open apice, a wait-and-see strategy is accepted due to the considerable potential of revascularization [87], which occurs in up to 100% of these teeth [81]. In such a case, endodontic treatment is performed only if signs of pulp necrosis or root resorption are detected [87]. On the other hand, some authors suggested a wait-and-see strategy even in cases with closed apices [88, 89]. In the study by Ahlberg et al. [89], 30% of 33 maxillary canines with complete root formation required no endodontic treatment after an average of 6 years. (Figure 1)

5. Surgical exposure of teeth and orthodontic treatment

The most desirable treatment approach for the management of impacted maxillary canines is early diagnosis and interception of potential impaction. However, in the absence of prevention, clinicians should consider surgical exposure and orthodontic alignment.

This treatment option is recommended when: [59]

a.   the patient tends to wear orthodontic appliances

b.   the patient is well motivated and has general good dental health

c.   the long axis of the ectopic canine is not too horizontal or oblique. The closer the crown is to the midline and the root to the mid-palatal suture, the poorer pronosis for alignment [60]

d.   any evidence of root resorption or other pathology is such that it is more desirable to preserve the canine. For instance if the adjacent lateral incisor is resorbed and have a very poor prognosis, it would be advantageous to attempt alignment of impacted canine to replace the lateral incisor [59].

Two approaches could be followed after surgical exposure: [21]

1.   surgical exposure to allow for natural eruption to occur

2.   surgical exposure with the placement of an auxiliary

8.1. Surgical exposure to allow for natural eruption to occur

This method is often used when:

• the canine has an appropriate axial inclination and does not need to be uprighted during its eruption,

- the root development has not been completed yet, therefore patient' s age is important

The progress of canine eruption should be monitored with roentgenograms, using reference points such as an adjacent tooth or the arch wire. If the tooth fails to erupt, removal of any cicatricial tissue surrounding the crown is recommended. The main disadvantages of this approach are the spontaneous but slow canine eruption, the increased treatment time, and the inability to influence the path of eruption and the risk of ankylosing [21].

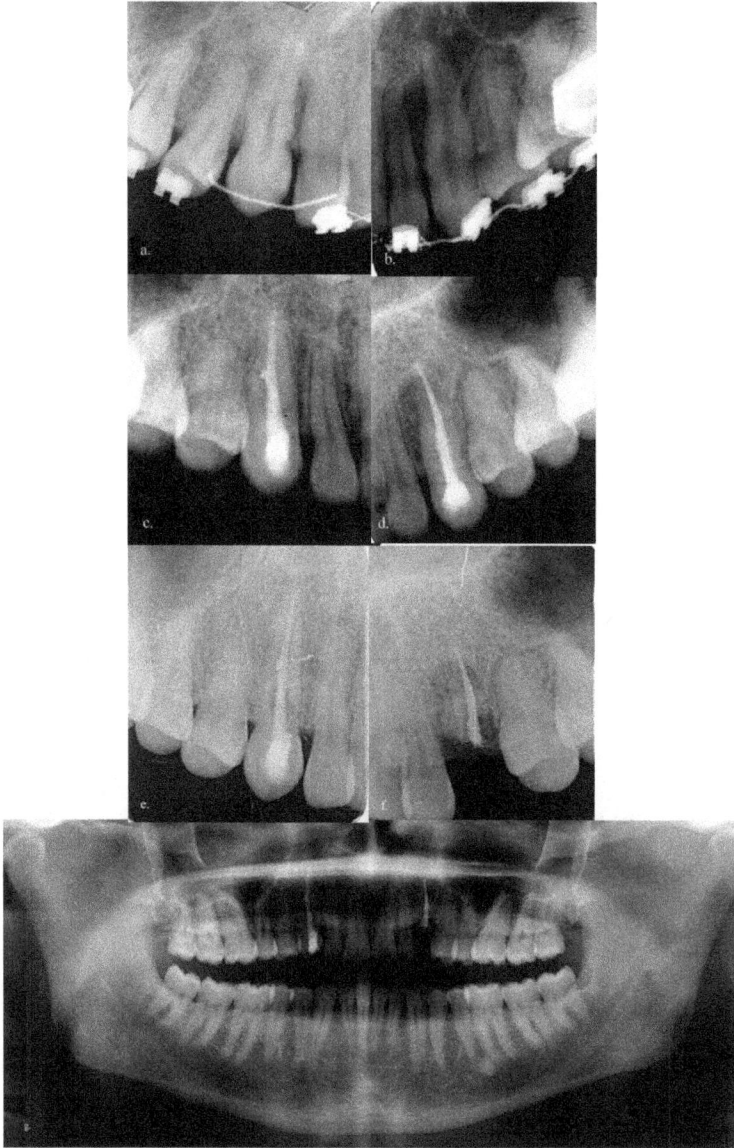

Figure 1. Bilateral impacted canines were treated with autotransplantation in a 22 year old adult patient. A wait and see strategy was followed and canal therapy was applied after seven months from autotransplantation as external root resorption was detected. 10 years after treatment the patient came with the left canine broken due to external root resorption, however no difference was observed in the contralateral canine.

8.2. Surgical exposure with the placement of an auxiliary

Surgically assisted orthodontic guidance is required when all possibilities of its natural eruption have been failed. It is preffered to be performed at least 6 months after root apex completion [10]. The duration of this orthodontic treatment varies from 12–36 months depending on a number of factors including the patient's age, crowding, the angulation and bucco-palatal position of the tooth, its distance from the occlusal plane and the periodontal health [8]. If the inclination of the canine is greater than 45 degrees in relation to the midline then the prognosis for alignment worsens. The further the canine needs to be moved then the poorer the diagnosis for a successful outcome. Either the tooth should not be anyklosed or the root not be dilaserated [60]. Correct root positioning and a good buccal overlap is necessary for a stable result [90]. The prognosis is worse in older patients than in young patients, thus early diagnosis is essential [42]. The upper age limits suggested for successful alignment of an unerupted canine are 16 and 20 years [57]. In contrast Nieri et al. [8] found the position of the impacted canines closer to the physiologic position of the dental arch in older subjects which affected the treatment duration positively.

Combined forced eruption treatment approach is performed at three phases [8].

- surgical exposure of the impacted tooth

- placement of an attachment to the tooth

- application of orthodontic mechanics to align the impacted teeth

Mostly two approaches are recommended in regards to the timing of attachment placement: [21]

1. The first method is a two-step approach. Firstly the canine is surgically uncovered and the area is packed with a surgical dressing in order to avoid filling in of tissues around the tooth. After wound healing within 3-8 weeks, the pack is removed, then an attachment is bonded on the impacted tooth [91]. This approach is preferred when bleeding compromises attachment bonding [92].

2. The second method is a one-step approach, in which, the attachment is placed on the tooth at the time of surgical exposure. This method is especially recommended for palatally impacted teeth which aids the clinician to visualize and better control the direction of tooth movement when traction force is applied.

8.3. Surgical exposure of the impacted tooth

During surgical exposure of an impacted tooth, only enough bone should be removed for the placement of a bonded bracket [21]. Excision of tissues must be carefully performed and the cementoenamel junction (CEJ) should not be intentionally exposed. If done incorrectly, the unerupted tooth may be left with inadequate keratinized tissue. Therefore the use of electro-surgical or laser techniques is contraindicated for surgical exposure. These instruments are designed for removal of hard and soft tissues, the contact of the instrument to the tooth may lead to permanent damage of either type of tissue and/or devitalization of the tooth [20].

Main indicator of the treatment success of impacted maxillary canines is related with the final periodontal outcome [49]. In earlier methods, radical bone was removed during surgical exposure and all bony obstacles were removed to provide an easier path for tooth eruption. Literature shows that the most serious periodontal damage is loss of supporting bone which is associated with more heavy surgical procedures involving exposure of the tooth underneath the cementoenamel junction (CEJ) [93]. Therefore exposure of the CEJ was a critical variable and special attention has to be given during surgery or when placing a wire lasso with or without a gold chain.

Classification and treatment techniques will be presented in detail according to the position of impacted maxillary canines:

8.4. Palatal versus labial impactions

The incidence rate of palatal impaction is at least 3:1 [94] and up to 6:1 when compared to labial impaction [95]. Labial impactions generally have a more favorable vertical angulation whereas palatally impacted canines are more often inclined in a horizontal/oblique direction [21]. Jacoby [32] determined that 85% of palatally impacted canines had enough space in the dental arch where as only 17% of the labially unerupted maxillary canines appeared to have sufficient space for eruption. Consequently he claimed arch length deficiency as a primary causative factor for labially impacted canines.

Ectopic labially positioned canines may erupt frequently high in the sulcus or alveolar ridge on their own without either surgical exposure or orthodontic treatment. Contrarily, palatally impacted canines seldom erupt without intervention due to the thickness of the palatal cortical bone and also the dense, thick, and resistant palatal mucosa [21].

8.5. Management of labially impacted canines

Labially impacted maxillary canine is often positioned high in the alveolar bone and erupts through the alveolar mucosa. It has been emphasized that labially impacted canines are more challenging to manage without the occurrence of adverse periodontal problems. Therefore, special attention has to be given to surgical technique, marginal gingival placement, control of inflammation, magnitude of force, atraumatic surgery, and proper gingival attachment [96].

Generally 3 techniques are used for uncovering a labially impacted maxillary canine [31]:

i.   excisional uncovering (gingivectomy)

ii.   apically positioned flap

iii.   closed eruption techniques

The orthodontist should guide the surgeon properly to select an appropriate technique. If the correct uncovering technique is chosen, the eruption process can be simplified, resulting in a predictably stable and esthetic result. Four criteria should be evaluated by the orthodontist in order to determine the appropriate method for uncovering the tooth before referring a patient for surgical exposure. First, the labiolingual position of the impacted canine crown should be determined. If the tooth is impacted labially, then any of the 3 techniques could be performed, since there is usually little or any bone covering the crown of the impacted canine. However, if the tooth is impacted in the center of the alveolus, an excisional approach and an apically positioned flap are usually more difficult to perform, for large amount of bone removal might be required from the labial surface of the crown.

The second criterion to evaluate is the vertical position of the tooth relative to the mucogingival junction. Any of the 3 techniques can be chosen to uncover the tooth, if most of the canine crown is positioned coronal to the mucogingival junction. (Figure 2)

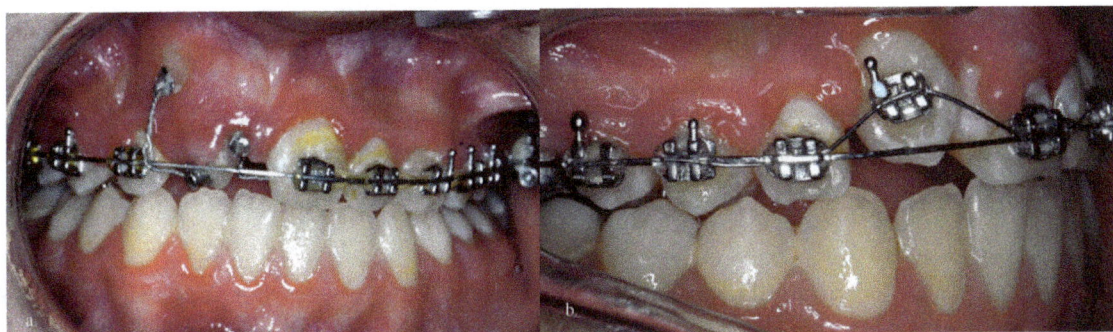

Figure 2. Closed flap technique was performed for the maxillary canine to erupt and orthodontic traction was applied to align the canine into the lateral position.

When the canine crown is positioned apical to the mucogingival junction, the most appropriate approach is the closed eruption technique for it would provide adequate gingiva over the crown and prevent reintrusion of the tooth in the long term [97]. Excisional technique would be inappropriate, because it would result in no gingiva over the labial surface of the tooth after eruption has completed. An apically positioned flap would either be inappropriate since it would cause possible reintrusion and instability of the crown of the tooth after orthodontic treatment [98].

The third criterion to evaluate is the amount of attached gingiva in the area of the impacted canine. The creation and preservation of the band of attached gingiva is very critical for periodontal health in the management of labially impacted teeth [12]. The only technique that predictably would produce more gingiva is an apically positioned flap, if there were insufficient gingiva in the area of the canine. Otherwise, mucogingival recession and alveolar bone loss may occur. Any of the 3 techniques could be selected, if there were sufficient gingiva to provide at least 2 to 3 mm of attached gingiva over the canine crown after it had been erupted [31].

The final criterion to evaluate is the mesiodistal position of the canine crown. An apically positioned flap should be preferred if the crown were positioned mesially and over the root of the lateral incisor, since it could be difficult to move the tooth through the alveolus unless it was completely exposed. In this situation, closed eruption or excisional uncovering generally would not be recommended [31].

There are conflicting reports in the literature regarding apically positioned flap technique and closed eruption technique [64,98-100]. Unfortunately, some reports and studies have failed to differentiate that the "open" technique is different from an apically positioned flap approach [96]. There is conclusive evidence that an open eruption approach through nonkeratinized gingival should be avoided [98]. The absence of an adequate band of attached gingiva around the erupting canine may cause inflammation of the periodontium. Vanarsdall and Corn [99] emphasized that it is risky to move teeth in the presence of inflammation. In addition Caprioglio et al. [101] stated that it is necessary to use conservative surgical techniques and orthodontic systems mimicking the natural pattern of eruption in order to achieve adequate periodontal status.

An apically repositioned flap or closed eruption techniques through keratinized gingival tissue are recommended [102]. If the tissue is too thin to be dissected as a partial thickness graft, laterally repositioned pedicle graft, a free gingival graft can be performed initially to increase the thickness of keratinized gingiva. After approximately 30 to 60 days or complete healing of the grafted tissue, the tooth may be exposed, bonded, and orthodontic traction might be applied.

Vernette et al. [98] compared the esthetic and periodontal results between the apically repositioned flap and the closed eruption techniques of surgically uncovering labially impacted maxillary teeth (incisors and canines). They have concluded that periodontal attachment differences between uncovered and contralateral teeth were not clinically significant in either the apically positioned flap or closed-eruption groups. However labially impacted maxillary anterior teeth uncovered with an apically positioned flap technique have more unesthetic sequalae than those with closed-eruption technique. Also adverse effects were detected treated with apically positioned flap technique such as increased clinical crown length, width of attached tissue, gingival scarring, and intrusive relapse since the mucosal attachment tends to pull the crown of the tooth apically.

However in literature the disadvantages of closed eruption technique were reported as increase in treatment time, additional surgical procedures, diminished control of tooth movement, as well as adverse periodontal responses [21,96]. Advantages of the apically positioned graft are that it is minimally invasive, provides controlled tooth movement (even high in the vestibular depth), prevents cystic follicles, decreases treatment time. Also it prevents ankylosis if bonding is delayed for 1 week [96]. It was reported that only 4 to 5 months was enough to erupt labially impacted teeth into the arch with apically positioned grafts even in severe cases [103].

In the review article of Vanarshdal [96] it was concluded that adverse responses have not been determined with labially uncovered teeth with grafts that have been left open and activated a week later. Surgical exposure with careful attention to the periodontal tissues and proper orthodontic alignment without intentional closing over with soft tissue could provide a more predictable result for patients. It was also emphasized that the pedicle graft is necessary on the labial of the maxilla. The gingivally repositioned procedure as described earlier [99] didn' t create a compromised periodontal outcome, and treated teeth were indistinguishable from untreated sides Vanarshdal [96] stated that closed eruption technique was not superior to apically repositioned flap technique as a result of this evidence based data.

Apart from these comman used three techniques explained above, the application of tunnel technique might be indicated in the following situations: [8]

i.   if persistent deciduous canines exists with impacted canines or space available in the dental arch and

ii.   feasibility of direct traction of the impacted canine to the center of the alveolar ridge as assessed on the diagnostic radiographic records to reproduce the physiologic eruption pattern of the canine.

8.6. Management of the palatally impacted canines

The most common impaction encountered by orthodontists is the palatal impaction of maxillary canines (95-Stellzig et al., 1994). With palatal impactions it is critical to recognize that the entire palate is covered with specialized mucosa and a graft is not necessary [104]. The most commonly used surgical methods for exposing the impacted canine are: [59]

1. open surgical exposure and allowing for natural eruption

2. open surgical exposure and packing with subsequent bonding of an auxillary

3. closed surgical exposure with the placement of an auxiliary attachment intraoperatively.

The first method is most appropriate if the canine has the correct inclination and will then erupt spontaneously. Schmidt [105] suggested to uncover palatally impacted canines early, during the mixed dentition in order to encourage autonomous eruption, without orthodontic intervention. They have reported that the overall treatment time is reduced with superior periodontal and aesthetic results since the bone levels and attachment levels improved on the canine and lateral incisor and also little to no root resorption occured on the lateral incisors.

Kokich and Mathews [100] also recommended earlier timing for uncovering palatally impact-ed canines before starting orthodontic treatment. In some cases, surgical exposure could be performed during the late mixed dentition. First a full-thickness mucoperiosteal flap is elevated, then all bone over the crown is removed down to the cementoenamel junction. Following the flap is returned, and a hole is made through the gingival flap. If the tooth is highly positioned in the palate a dressing might be placed over the exposed area in the flap. Although it has been noted that autonomous eruption occurs within 6 to 9 months postoper-atively, there is currently no report in the literature to support this statement [106]. After the canines erupt to the occlusal level an attachment could be bonded for the further orthodontic treatment.

The second approach is the "open window" eruption technique in which a flap is elevated and enough amount of bone is removed to expose the tip of the impacted crown to be bonded. The flap is then repositoned and sutured with a small "window" cut into the flap of the palatal soft tissue, covering the embedded crown packed with surgical dressing. To provide a good periodontal prognosis, a special attention should be given in maintaining the attached gingiva on the impacted tooth. One week later postoperatively the pack is removed and an attachment is bonded with subsequent traction using a fixed appliance. There is some evidence that the periodontal status may be compromized [107]. (Figure 3)

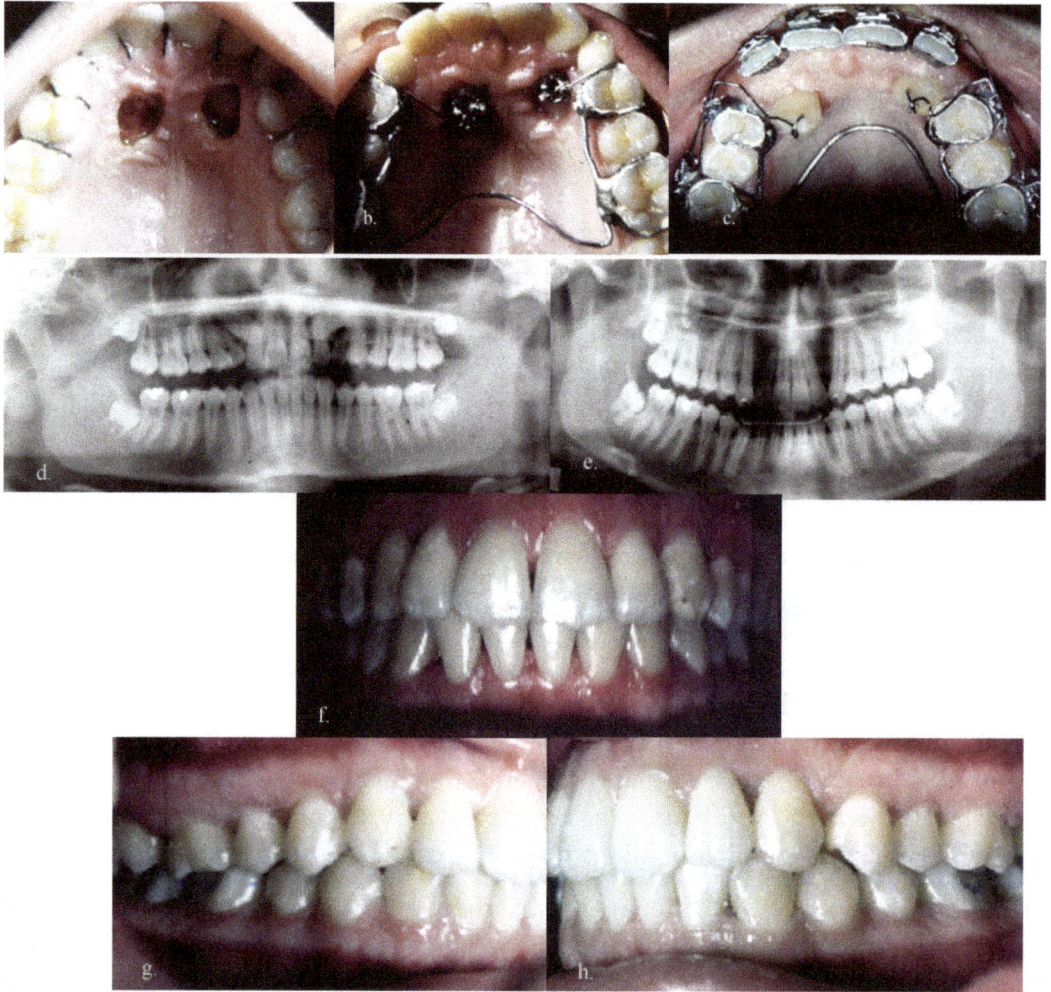

Figure 3. Bilateral palatally impacted maxillary canines were uncovered by open surgical technique, orthodontic traction was performed by ballista springs. Alignment of bilateral maxillary canines lasted 4,5 years.

The third option is the closed eruption technique. If a canine is associated with severe resorption of the root of the incisor, an open exposure is not indicated since it endangers the vitality and existence of the incisor. In such a case a closed eruption technique would provide both teeth a vital state [108]. In this technique sufficient space should be created before the surgical exposure. Usually uncovering a palatally impacted canine occurs after the first 6 to 9 months of orthodontic alignment of the maxillary dentition. In this technique firstly a mucoperiostal flap is reflected and a minimum of bone is removed to reveal the follicle,which is opened at the most superficial point only. Bone is not cleared away from the neck of the tooth, nor more of the follicular tissue than is essential for bonding, and certainly not down to the cementoenamel junction [109]. A small eyelet, threaded with soft twisted ligature wire of 0.012-in gauge, is then bonded while hemostasis is maintained. The flap is then sutured fully back to cover the entire wound and exposed area, with the twisted ligature wire drawn through the flap at a point strategically placed to permit traction in the direction that will have been confirmed when the orthodontist actually sees the tooth in situ. Generally, orthodontic traction begins soon after the surgery towards to the edentulous site [109].

On the other hand if not enough bone is removed then the tooth will not move and orthodontist might suspect from anyklosis. However the incidence of ankylosed maxillary canines is low [100]. In the case of insufficient bone removal over the impacted tooth, the tooth will not be able to resorb the bone over the crown efficiently for the dental follicle is deflated and removed. When a force is applied the enamel of the impacted crown comes into contact with the bone however there are no cells in the enamel to resorb the bone. Therefore resorption will eventually occur slowly through pressure necrosis [31].

Closed eruption technique is a more conservative approach however if bond failure occurs then re-exposure is required. Also direct bonding of the impacted canine during surgery may cause soft tissue injury due to the acid etching contamination. Becker et al. [108] suggested the use of an eyelet bonded in a mid-buccal position on the crown of the impacted tooth at surgery as these have the highest success rate. Becker and Chausu [109] stated that morbidity is lower in closed eruption approach than for open procedures since healing is faster, postoperative pain is considerably reduced, and postsurgical bleeding is virtually eliminated.

There is a controversy in the literature regarding the periodontal outcome of open or closed surgical exposure and subsequent orthodontic alignment of the palatally displaced canines [110]. It is believed that periodontal health is compromised when the palatal mucosa is excised with open technique [93].) However in a systematic review Parkin et al. [111] found no robust evidence to support one surgical technique over the other.

Also in recent studies [112, 113] evaluating the differences in the periodontal outcomes of palatally displaced canines (PDC) exposed with either an open or a closed surgical technique, no significant differences in post-treatment periodontal status of the canines and adjacent teeth were determined between the techniques. Both treatment methods were found acceptable for treatment of the palatally impacted canine. In addition Smailine et al., [113] 2013 concluded that post-treatment periodontal status and the level of bone support were not dependent on the patients' age at the start of treatment, the duration of treatment, or the initial horizontal and vertical localization of impacted canine.

9. Orthodontic considerations

Orthodontic treatment methodology for impacted canines depends on various factors, such as location of the impacted canine in the dental arch relative to adjacent incisors, the distance from the occlusal plane, canine crown overlaps, canine angulations, the possible presence of ankylosis, root resorption, or dilaceration [100]. Generally, horizontally impacted or ankylosed canines are the most hazardous to manage and have the poorest prognosis [114]. Some of these teeth may need to be extracted. These variables are also used as predictors of the orthodontic treatment duration [100].

Frequently, when the palatally impacted canine is surgically uncovered, only the lingual surface of the tooth is available for bonding attachments. However Becker and coworkers [107] stated that the palatal surface as the poorest bonding surface. The orthodontic force to be applied to the bonded attachment requires careful planning because if an orthodontic force is applied from the adjacent maxillary teeth, it will tend to embed the buccal surface of the crown and may create periodontal problems. In order to prevent this problem, first the tooth should be erupted vertically and once a facial attachment can be bonded, forces should direct the tooth facially [115].

When removal of premolars is planned for the orthodontic treatment, it is advised to delay their extractions until the canine is surgically uncovered and feasibility of moving the impacted canine is insured. However, the premolar has to be removed initially prior to any attempt to move the canine in severely crowded cases. In such a case, the patient or parents should be made aware of the possible complications [21].

During closed-eruption technique, the orthodontist should select mechanics that erupt the tooth through the center of the alveolar ridge. The eruption of the tooth between the alveolar cortical plates prevents bone dehiscence and unfavorable orthodontic and esthetic consequences [49]. The mechanics that draw the tooth labially should be avoided, in order not to produce a bony dehiscence or labial recession of gingival magrin [31].

The impacted tooth under orthodontic traction forces should be periodically checked for excessive mobility or bleeding from gingiva around the tooth. It is important to ensure that periodontal attachment is following the tooth as it is guided into the arch [116]. Furthermore correction of torque, labio-palatal root angulation of the impacted canine should be considered to achieve proper functional occlusion. The bracket on the labial aspect of the canine can be inverted to correct the torque or a mandibular premolar bracket can bonded to the ectopic canine to produce a more negative torque [117].

9.1. Methods of attachment

Wire ligatures, a bracket, a hook, button or an eyelet directly may be attached to the enamel surface after the surgical exposure of the impacted tooth crown [29]. (Figure 2,3) If the canines are deeply impacted, a gold chain may be used that can pass through a long tunnel created between the impacted tooth and the empty socket of the extracted primary canine [118]. A circumferential, dead soft, ligature wire (lasso) passing around the cervical area of the tooth shouldn' t be used as an attachment since too much bone removal is required. This "heavy exposure," may provoke the risk of injuring the adjacent teeth, external root resorption and ankylosis [119]. Celli et al. [120] advocated bonding of two attachments to the impacted canine instead of the classic single one for closed eruption of palatally impacted canines in order to reduce the potential risk of a second surgical operation when the traction attachment comes off.

9.2. Traction methods

Various methods have been used for moving the canine into proper alignment. These include the use of light wires (Figure 2) or springs soldered to a heavy labial or palatal base wire, mousetrap loops, K-9 spring, ballista loops (Figure 3c), Kilroy I, II springs [31, 121, 122]. Vardimon et al. [123] recommended the use of magnets to treat impacted canines on the basis of a less invasive surgical procedure, effective forces at short distances, and controlled spatial guidance. (Figure 4) With the introduction of new orthodontic materials such as elastic threads, elastometric chains, and nickeltitanium springs, the orthodontist has a wider choice of materials and also greater control of the force magnitude and direction.

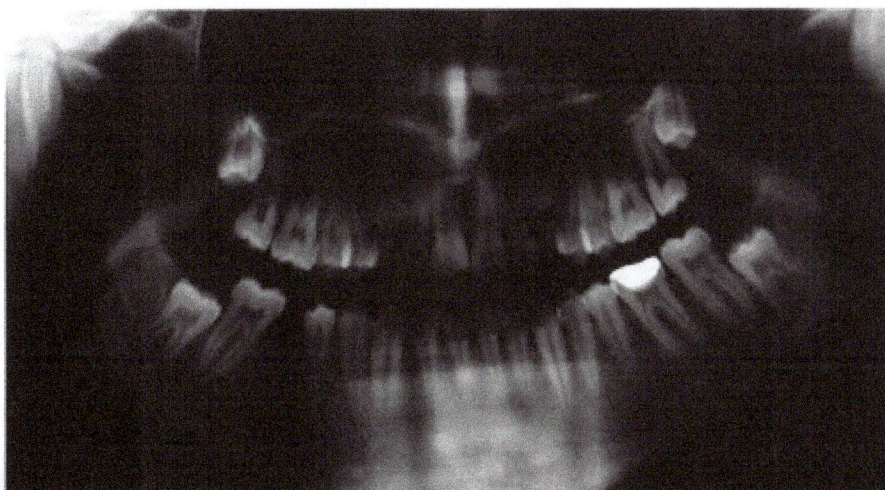

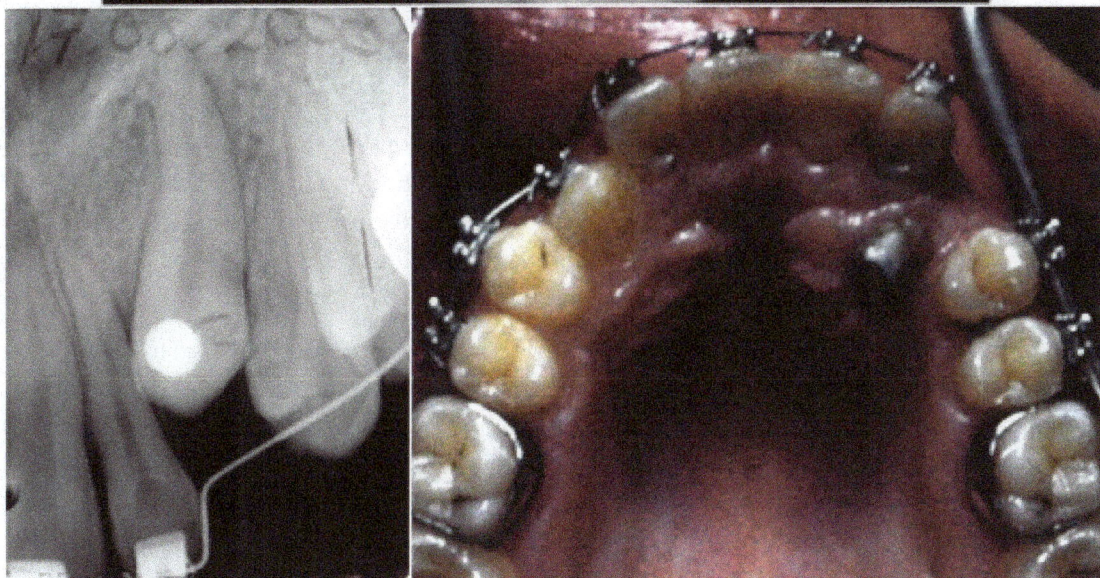

Figure 4. Orthodontic traction of bilateral impacted canines with the use of magnets. Right maxillary canine closer to the surface could be erupted with magnets. The left canine also moved closer along the top of the arch, however the patient discontinued his treatment.

An efficient way to make impacted canines erupt is to use closed-coil springs with eyelets, as long as no obstacles impede the path of the canine. If the canine is in close proximity to the incisor roots and a buccally directed force is applied, then it will contact the roots of adjacent teeth and may cause damage. (Figure 5) In addition, the canine position may not improve due to the root obstacle. Therefore regardless of the material used, the direction of the applied force should initially move the impacted tooth away from the roots of the neighboring teeth. In addition, the following is recommended: [21]

1. Initially maxillary arch should be levelled and aligned until a rigid rectangular arch can be inserted prior to the surgical exposure of the impacted tooth and application of traction forces [115].

2. Enough space should either be available in the arch or should be created for the impacted tooth;

3. In order to preserve the space created, either continuously tie the teeth mesially and distally to the canine or place a close coiled spring on the arch wire;

4. The eruption path might require the fabrication of auxiliaries numerous times due to anatomic obstructions during the traction process to redirect forces [115].

5. The use of light forces to move the impacted tooth, no more than 2 oz (60 g);

6. The arch wire should have enough stiffness, such as.018 ×.022, to resist deformation against traction forces during canine extrusion (Figure 2). The added stiffness of the arch wire will diminsh the undesirable "rollercoaster" effect caused by intrusion of the neighboring anchor teeth as a reaction to the deflection of a lighter and hence more flexible arch wire. Therefore, the magnitude of the force applied should not deflect the arch wire.

Orthodontic traction on the impacted tooth should be applied with light forces (20 to 30 g). In most of the cases, the root tip of the impacted canine is usually in a good position, so a tipping movement (light movement) is appropriate to move the crown toward the dental arch. The combined effects of "light" surgical exposure, "light" orthodontic movements, and "light" orthodontic forces are beneficial to the future periodontal health of the tooth since they minimize the loss of alveolar bone support and potential injury to the tooth during traction. However "heavy movement" such as torque during the traction cause more bone loss [21].

Fixed or removable appliances can be used for the traction of impacted tooth. However there are certain disadvantages of removable appliances such as the need for patient cooperation, limited control of tooth movement, and the inability to treat complex malocclusions [21] therefore only in cases with multiple missing teeth Hawley-type appliances might be used which transfer anchorage demands to the palatal vault and the alveolar ridge [124].

Most techniques have used the maxillary arch as anchorage for traction, which may be unsuitable in many clinical situations [94]. In cases in which the impacted canine is situated palatal to the lateral incisor, firstly an attempt should be made to move the canine away from lateral incisor before moving the impacted tooth toward the dental arch. In this situation if the desired forces cannot be applied from within the maxillary arch, mandibular arch might be

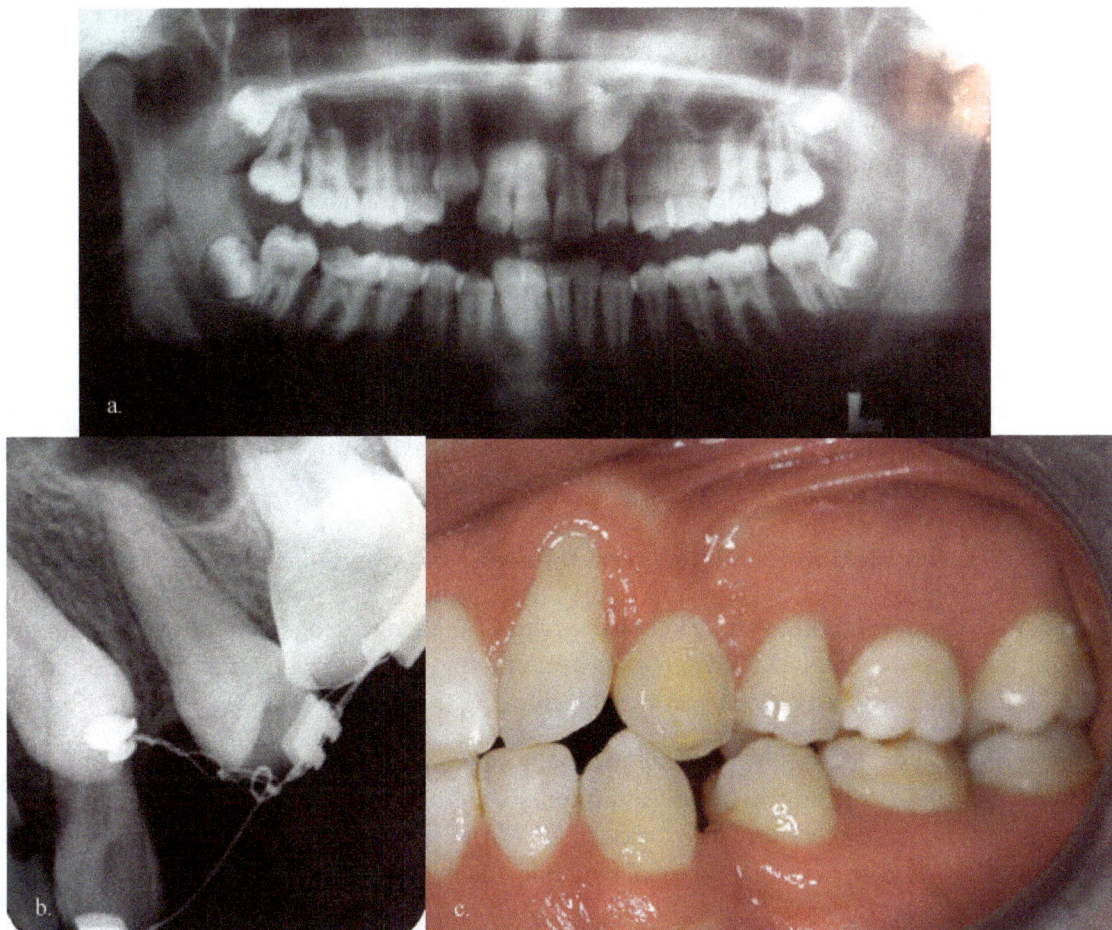

Figure 5. A buccally directed traction of a palatally impacted maxillary canine resulted in the buccal movement of the adjacent lateral root due to the close approximity and gingival recession was observed 10 years after treatment.

used as a source of anchorage. A mandibular fixed lingual arch with a vertical hook can be used for this purpose. Elastics are engaged in these vertical hooks and to the attachment on the impacted teeth for the required traction. In addition directional forces can be used by applying elastics. The main disadvantege of mandibular anchorage is the difficulty encountered in controlling the magnitude and direction of the applied forces because of the mobile mandibular arch [115].

Recently mini-screws have been proved to be reliable and convenient skeletal anchorage devices in the management of unerupted canines. Their mechanical resistance was found suitable for the initial orthodontic traction of these teeth. Mini-screws are placed in the alveolar process to improve the initial angulation of impacted canine teeth. Following soft tissue healing around the exposed tooth, mechanical traction can be activated with a nickel-titanium closed-coil spring exerting gentle forces 0.5–0.8 N (50–80 g) of force. The main advantage of this method is that the maxillary arch should not be bracketed until the canine has begun to move and ankylosis can be ruled out [125].

Poggio et al. [126] studied the interradicular anatomy of 25 patients with volumetric tomographic imaging. On the palatal side, the most available bone was determined between the second premolar and first molar whereas on the buccal side between the two premolars. These areas were found convenient for the clinical application of a mini-screw if extrusion of a palatally impacted canine is planned. On the buccal side less bone was determined between the second premolar and first molar. On the palatal side, the interseptal distance between the two molars was either less, yet still sufficient.

Impacted teeth tend to respond much later in adults than do those in children. Chaushu et al. [127] advised the placement of a temporary anchorage device in the palate at the time of closed exposure and the immediate application of elastic traction for several months since they have experienced failure of teeth to erupt despite the application of traction in patients in their fourth and fifth decades of life. They place orthodontic appliances if positive signs of movement are observed.

9.3. Retention considerations and long term follow-up of impacted canines

Treatment of impacted tooth is almost always a clinical challenge. Holistic treatment planning, prudent flap design, coupled with forced eruption using light extrusive forces, periodontal health and functional occlusion are central to achieving the desired long-term results.

Becker et al. [128] evaluated the posttreatment alignment of the impacted canines in patients who had completed their orthodontic treatment. They observed an increased incidence of rotations or spacings on the "impacted" side in 17.4% of the cases, whereas on the control side the incidence was only 8.7%. The control side had ideal alignment twice as often as did the impacted side.

Capriogli et al. [101] evaluated the long-term (4.6 years) periodontal response of palatally impacted maxillary canines aligned using a closed-flap surgical technique in association with a codified orthodontic traction system. No damage to periodontium was detected in the long-term.

Woloshyn et al. [129] evaluated the posttreatment changes nearly 4 years after treatment and compared the differences in the periodontal and pulpal status, root length, and tooth alignment between the side of the forced-erupted ectopically canine and the contralateral side. The probing attachment level was found lower on the mesial and distal aspect of the previously impacted canines, also the roots of the adjacent teeth were found shorter. The incidance of pulpal obliteration was 21% in the previously impacted canines. Significant posttreatment changes such as intrusion, lingual displacement, rotation, and discoloration was determined in 40% of the previously impacted teeth where as 91% had a normal appearance on the contralateral side.

A fiberotomy or a bonded fixed retainer is suggested to prevent rotational relapse, after the completion of the desired movements and often before the appliances are removed. Removing a "halfmoon-shaped wedge" of tissue from the lingual side of the canine might intercept lingual drift after correction of palatally impacted canines [130].

D'Amico et al. [131] reported the adverse effects of the orthodontic-surgical treatment for impacted maxillary canines in the long term conducted in a sample of 61 cases. 6.5% of the patients were dissatisfied with the esthetic results, whereas the orthodontist estimated the results as good in only 57% of the cases. Canine guidance was detected less frequently on the working side during lateral movements in previously impacted canines due to the significant difference in their inclination compared to normally erupted ones.

9.4. Frequent complications observed with unerupted teeth

Surgical exposure of the impacted tooth and the complex orthodontic mechanisms that are applied to align the impacted tooth into the arch may lead to deleterious consequences for the supporting structures of the tooth, such as displacement and devitalization, ankylosis or loss of vitality, recurrent pain, cystic degeneration, invasive servical root resorption, external root resorption of the canine and adjacent teeth. Furthermore loss of periodontal bone support, gingival recession, sensitivity problems or combinations of these factors may be observed [129].(Figure 5) Most of these risks can be prevented with proper management of periodontal tissues and timing of care. These problems can result in prolonged treatment time, esthetic deformities and often the loss of teeth.

If no movement of the impacted canine is observed, this may be as a result of single or combination of the following reasons: [132]

• inappropriate positional diagnosis of the impacted teeth and its relationship with the roots of the adjacent teeth which leads to incorrect direction of traction

• a lack of considerably anchorage requirement will lead to inefficient mechanotherapy and unnecassarily longer treatment

• anyklosis might have afflicted the impacted tooth either a priori or as the result of the earlier surgical or the orthodontic maneuers.

• scar tissue might have blocked the wire chain, [133]

If, the tooth does not show clear evidence of movement after six months of orthodontic force application, a re-evaluation is necessary. Ankylosis, one of the major complications associated with impacted canines, can rarely be detected based on clinical and conventional radiographic examinations however CBCT provides a better diagnosis of the area of ankylosis [134].

In the recent study of Koutzoglou and Kostaki [135] evidence of an association between exposure technique and ankylosis was determined. The percentage of ankylosis was 3.5% in the open technique and 14.5% in the closed technique. They have defined anyklosis as impacted canines being immobilized a priori or during traction, due to all the possible causes that could contribute to immobilization, such as all types of external tooth resorption and other known or unknown factors. Additionally, they found a evidence that the grade of impaction and the patient's age are significant predictors of ankylosis.

Traditionally, once a tooth becomes ankylosed, surgical luxation has been the treatment of choice [136]. Although orthodontic light forces are applied immediately after luxation to prevent reankylosis, ankylosis often occurs again [137]. Another viable treatment option for ankylosed or dilacerated maxillary canines is apicotomy proposed by Puricelli [138] in 1987. An apicotomy is a guided fracture of a canine root apex performed with a small chisel followed by orthodontic traction of the canine crown. Puricelli's data [138, 139] showed that in 29 patients who had the procedure, 26 procedures were successful and 3 failed.

Becker and Chausu [109] stated that invasive cervical root resorption is the cause of many failed impacted teeth, rather than the knee-jerk and usually unproven application of the label "ankylosis." It is difficult to diagnose on a radiograph, yet, as the lesion grows, bone is usually deposited in the depth of the resorption lacunae, and then the tooth will no longer respond to extrusive traction [140]. Radical surgery extending down to the cementoenamel junction is likelihood of this possible sequel.

Becker et al. [132] reported that repeat surgery was required for 62.9% of the impacted canines in which corrective treatment was started, mostly to redirect the ligature wires with the guidance of the 3-dimensional imaging. If orthodontic traction fails other treatment options should be considered. Prosthetic replacement might be performed yet preparation of the adjacent, usually healthy teeth for a conventional fixed bridge is far from ideal. Implant placement would be another option that generally requires extraction of the impacted tooth. However this causes a bony defect which must be bone-grafted. Orthodontic closure of the gap might also be considered but it results in asymmetry in unilateral cases [125].

10. Conclusions

The management of impacted canines is important in terms of esthetics and function and, requires a qualified experience of a number of clinicians. If patients are evaluated and treated appropriately, then the frequency of ectopic eruption and subsequent impaction of the maxillary canine can be reduced. Various surgical and orthodontic techniques may be used to uncover impacted maxillary canines related to its position. Accurate localization, conservative management of the soft tissues, selection of appropriate surgical approach, rigid anchorage unit, and the direction of the orthodontic traction are the important factors for the successful management of impacted canines.

Author details

Belma Işık Aslan* and Neslihan Üçüncü

*Address all correspondence to: belmaslan2003@yahoo.com

Gazi University, Faculty of Dentistry, Department of Orthodontics, Ankara, Turkey

References

[1] Lindauer SJ, Rubenstein LK, Hang WM, Andersen WC, Isaacson RJ. Canine Impaction Identified Early with Panoramic Radiographs. The Journal of American Dental Association 1992;123(3) 91–92.

[2] Litsas G, Acar A. A Review of Early Displaced Maxillary Canines: Etiology, Diagnosis and Interceptive Treatment. The Open Dentistry Journal 2011; 5: 39-47.

[3] Brin I, Becker A, Shalhav M. Position of the Maxillary Permanent Canine in Relation to Anomalous or Missing Lateral Incisors: a Population Study. European Journal of Orthodontics 1986; 8(1) 12-16.

[4] Chu FC, Li TK, Lui VK, Newsome PR, Chow RL, Cheung LK. Prevalence of Impacted Teeth and Associated Pathologies-a Radiographic Study of the Hong Kong Chinese Population. Hong Kong Medical Journal 2003; 9(3) 158-163.

[5] Thilander B, Myrberg N. The Prevalence of Malocclusion in Swedish School Children. Scandinavian Journal of Dental Research 1973; 81(1) 12-21.

[6] Johnston WD. Treatment of Palatally Impacted Canine Teeth. American Journal of Orthodontics 1969; 56(6) 589-596.

[7] Ericson S, Kurol J. Resorption of Incisors After Ectopic Eruption of Maxillary Canines. A CT study. Angle Orthodontist 2000; 70(6) 415-423.

[8] Nieri M, Crescini A, Rotundo R, Baccetti T, Cortellini P, Pini Prato GP. Factors Affecting the Clinical Approach to Impacted Maxillary Canines: a Bayesian Network Analysis. American Journal of Orthodontics and Dentofacial Orthopedics 2010; 137(6) 755-762.

[9] Ericson S, Kurol J. Radiographic Examination of Ectopically Erupting Maxillary Canines. American Journal of Orthodontics and Dentofacial Orthopedics 1988; 91(6) 483-492.

[10] Coulter J, Richardson A. Normal Eruption of the Maxillary Canine Quantified in Three Dimensions. European Journal of Orthodontics 1997; 19(2) 171–183.

[11] Van Der Linden PGM. Transition of the Human Dentition. Monograph, Craniofacial Growth Series. Ann Arbor, MI, Center For Human Growth And Development: University Of Michigan;1982

[12] Becker A. The Orthodontic Treatment Of Impacted Teeth 2nd Ed. Jerusalem: Informa Healthcare; 2007.

[13] Moyers RE, Van Der Linden FP, Riolo ML, Mcnamara Jr. Standards of Human Occlusal Development. Monograph 5, Craniofacial Growth Series. Ann Arbor, MI, Center For Human Growth And Development: The University Of Michigan; 1976.

[14] Nanda SK. The Developmental Basis of Occlusion And Malocclusion. Chicago, IL: Quintessence Publishing; 1983.

[15] Roberts-Harry D, Sandy J. Orthodontics. Part 10: Impacted Teeth. British Dental Journal 2004; 196(6) 319–327.

[16] Brand RW, Isselhard DE. Anatomy of Orofacial Structures. 3rd Ed. St. Louis, MO: CV Mosby; 1986.

[17] Hurme VO. Ranges of Normalcy in the Eruption of Permanent Teeth. Jounal of Dentistry for Children 1949; 16(2) 11-15.

[18] Wise GE, King GJ. Mechanisms of Tooth Eruption and Orthodontic Tooth Movement. Journal of Dental Research 2008; 87(5) 414-434.

[19] Suri L, Gagari E, Vastardis H. Delayed Tooth Eruption: Pathogenesis, Diagnosis, and Treatment. A Literature Review. American Journal of Orthodontics and Dentofacial Orthopedics 2004; 126(4) 432-445.

[20] Ngan P, Hornbrook R, Weaver B. Early Timely Management of Ectopically Erupting Maxillary Canines. Seminars in Orthodontics 2005; 11: 152–163.

[21] Bishara SE. Clinical Management of Impacted Maxillary Canines. Seminars in Orthodontics 1998; 4(2) 87-98.

[22] Yawaka Y, Kaga M, Osanai M, Fukui A, Oguchi H. Delayed Eruption of Premolars with Periodontitis of Primary Predecessors and a Cystic Lesion: A Case Report. International Journal of Paediatric Dentistry 2002; 12(1) 53-60.

[23] Acquavella FJ. Delayed Eruption. Why? The New York State Dental Journal 1965; 31(10) 448-449.

[24] Tomizawa M, Yonemochi H, Kohno M, Noda T. Unilateral Delayed Eruption of Maxillary Permanent First Molars: Four Case Reports. Pediatric Dentistry 1998; 20(1) : 53-56.

[25] Katz J, Guelmann M, Barak S. Hereditary Gingival Fibromatosis with Distinct Dental, Skeletal and Developmental Abnormalities.Pediatric Dentistry 2002; 24(3) 253-256.

[26] Sekletov GA. Supercomplect Retained Tooth is the Cause of Delayed Eruption of the Upper Central Left Incisor. Therapy Stomatologiia 2001; 80(4) 66-68.

[27] Proffit WR, Vig KWL. Primary Failure of Eruption: A Possible Cause of Posterior Open-Bite. American Journal of Orthodontics and Dentofacial Orthopedics 1981;80(2) 173-190.

[28] Raghoebar GM, Boering G, Vissink A, Stegenga B. Eruption Disturbances of Permanent Molars: A Review. Journal of Oral Pathology & Medicine 1991; 20(4) 159-166.

[29] Bishara SE. Impacted Maxillary Canines: A Review. American Journal of Orthodontics and Dentofacial Orthopedics 1992; 101(2) 159-171.

[30] Pirinen S, Arte S, Apajalahti S. Palatal Displacement of Canine is Genetic and Related to Congenital Absence of Teeth. Journal of Dental Research 1996; 75(10) 1742-1746.

[31] Kokich VG. Surgical and Orthodontic Management of Impacted Maxillary Canines. American Journal of Orthodontics and Dentofacial Orthopedics 2004; 126(3) 278-283.

[32] Jacoby H. The Etiology Of Maxillary Canine Impactions. American Journal of Orthodontics 1983; 84(2) 125–132.

[33] Al-Nimri K, Gharaibeh T. Space Conditions and Dental and Occlusal Features in Patients with Palatally Impacted Maxillary Canines: An Aetiological Study. European Journal of Orthodontics 2005; 27(5) 461–465.

[34] Mcconnell TL, Hoffman DL, Forbes DP, Jensen EK, Wientraub NH. Maxillary Canine Impaction in Patients With Transverse Maxillary Deficiency. Journal of Dentistry for Children 1996; 63(3) 190–195.

[35] Langberg BJ, Peck S. Adequacy of Maxillary Dental Arch Width In Patients with Palatally Displaced Canines. American Journal of Orthodontics and Dentofacial Orthopedics 2000; 118(2) 220–223.

[36] Peck S, Peck L, Kataja M. Site-Specificity of Tooth Maxillary Agenesis in Subjects with Canine Malpositions. Angle Orthodontist 1996; 66(6) 473-476.

[37] Peck S, Peck L, Kataja M. Concomitant Occurrence of Canine Malposition and Tooth Agenesis: Evidence of Orofacial Genetic Fields. American Journal of Orthodontics and Dentofacial Orthopedics 2002; 122(6) 657-660.

[38] Sacerdoti R, Baccetti T. Dentoskeletal Features Associated With Unilateral Or Bilateral Palatal Displacement Of Maxillary Canines. Angle Orthodontist 2004; 74(6) 725-32.

[39] Shafer WG, Hine MK, Levy BM, Editors. A Textbook Of Oral Pathology. 2nd Ed. Philadelphia: WB Saunders; 1963.

[40] Suri L, Gagari E, Vastardis H. Delayed Tooth Eruption: Pathogenesis, Diagnosis, and Treatment. A Literature Review. American Journal of Orthodontics and Dentofacial Orthopedics 2004; 126(4) 432-445.

[41] Moss JP. The Unerupted Canine. The Dental Practitioner and Dental Record 1972; 22(6) 241-248.

[42] Ericson S, Kurol J. Longitudinal Study and Analysis of Clinical Supervision of Maxillary Canine Eruption. Community Dent Oral Epidemiol Community Dentistry and Oral Epidemiology 1986; 14(3) 172-176.

[43] Ericson S, Kurol J: Radiographic Assessment Of Maxillary Canine Eruption In Children with Clinical Signs of Eruption Disturbances. European Journal of Orthodontics 1981; 8(3) 133-140.

[44] Williams BHJ. Diagnosis and Prevention of Maxillary Cuspid Impaction. Angle Orthodontist 1981; 51(1) 30-40.

[45] Bishara SE. Clinical Management of Impacted Maxillary Canines. Seminars in Orthodontics 1998; 4(2) 87-98.

[46] Langland OE, Francis SH, Langlois RD. Atlas Of Special Technics in Dental Radiology. In: Textbook of Dental Radiology. Springfield, IL: Charles C. Thomas Publishes; 1984.

[47] Ericson S, Kurol J. Radiographic Examination of Ectopically Erupting Maxillary Canines. American Journal of Orthodontics and Dentofacial Orthopedics 1987; 91(6) 483-492.

[48] Turk MH, Katzenell J. Panoramic Localization. Oral Surgery, Oral Medicine and Oral Pathology 1970; 29(2) 212-215.

[49] Crescini A, Nieri M, Buti J, Baccetti T, Pini Prato GP. Pre-Treatment Radiographic Features for the Periodontal Prognosis of Treated Impacted Canines. Journal of Clinical Periodontology 2007; 34(7) 581-587.

[50] Liu DG, Zhang WL, Zhang ZY, Wu YT, Ma XC. Localization of Impacted Maxillary Canines and Observation of Adjacent Incisor Resorption with Cone-Beam Computed Tomography. Oral Surgery, Oral Medicine and Oral Pathology, Oral Radiology and Endodontics 2008; 105(1) 91-98.

[51] Boeddinghaus R, Whyte A. Current Concepts In Maxillofacial Imaging. European Journal of Radiology 2008; 66(3) 396-418.

[52] Alqerban A, Jacobs R, Keirsbilck P, Aly M, Swinnen S, Fieuws S, Willems G. The Effect of Using CBCT In the Diagnosis of Canine Impaction and Its Impact on the Orthodontic Treatment Outcome. Journal of Orthodontic Science. 2014; 3(2) 34–40.

[53] Wriedt S, Jaklin J, Al-Nawas B, Wehrbein H. Impacted Upper Canines: Examination and Treatment Proposal Based On 3D Versus 2D Diagnosis. Journal of Orofacial Orthopedics 2011; 73(1) 28-40.

[54] Alqerban A, Jacobs R, Lambrechts P, Loozen G, Willems G. Root Resorption of the Maxillary Lateral Incisor Caused by Impacted Canine: A Literature Review. Clinical Oral Investigations 2009; 13(3) 247-255.

[55] Oberoi S, Knueppel S. Three-Dimensional Assessment of Impacted Canines and Root Resorption Using Cone Beam Computed Tomography. Oral Surgery Oral Medicine Oral Pathology and Oral Radiology 2012; 113(2) 260-267.

[56] Taylor RW. Eruptive Abnormalities In Orthodontic Treatment. Seminars in Orthodontics 1998; 4(2) 79-86.

[57] Mc Sherry PF. The Assessment of and Treatment Options for the Burried Maxillary Canine. Dental Update 1996; 23(1) 7-10.

[58] Machen DE. Legal Aspects of Orthodontic Practice:Risk Management Concepts. The Impacted Canine. American Journal of Orthodontics and Dentofacial Orthopedics 1989; 96(3) 270-271.

[59] Mc Sherry PF. The Ectopic Maxillary Canine: A Review. British Journal of Orthodontics 1998; 25(3) 209-216.

[60] Kurol J, Ericson S, Andreasen JO. The Impacted Maxillary Canine. In: Andreasen JO, Kølsen Petersen J, Laskin D (eds.) Textbook And Color Atlas Of Tooth Impactions. Copenhagen: Munksgaard; 1997. p124-164.

[61] Ericson S, Kurol J. Early Treatment of Palatally Erupting Maxillary Canines by Extraction of the Primary Canines. European Journal of Orthodontics 1988; 10(4) 283-295.

[62] Power SM, Short MB. An Investigation into the Response of Palatally Displaced Canines to the Removal of Deciduous Canines and an Assessment of Factors Contributing to a Favourable Eruption. British Journal of Orthodontics 1993; 20(3) 215-223.

[63] Baccetti T, Leonardi M, Armi P. A Randomized Clinical Study of Two Interceptive Approaches to Palatally Displaced Canines. European Journal of Orthodontics 2008; 30(4) 381–385.

[64] Olive RJ. Orthodontic Treatment of Palatally Impacted Maxillary Canines. Australian Journal of Orthodontics 2002; 18(2) 64-70.

[65] Broadbent BH. Ontogenic Development of Occlusion. Angle Orthodontist 1941; 11(4) 223-241.

[66] Baccetti T, Sigler LM, Mcnamara JA. An RCT on Treatment of Palatally Displaced Canines with RME and/or a Transpalatal Arch. European Journal of Orthodontics 2011; 33(6) 601–607.

[67] Puricelli E, Morganti MA, Azambuja HV, Ponzoni D, Friedrisch CC. Partial Maxillary Osteotomy Following an Unsuccessful Forced Eruption of an Impacted Maxillary Canine-10 Year Follow-Up. Review and Case Report. Journal of Applied Oral Science 2012; 20(6) 667-72.

[68] Mirabella D, Giunta G, Lombardol. Substitution of Impacted Canines by Maxillary First Premolars: A Valid Alternative to Traditional Orthodontic Treatment. American Journal of Orthodontics and Dentofacial Orthopedics 2013; 143(1) 125-33.

[69] Rosa M, Zachrisson B. Integrating Space Closure and Esthetic Dentistry In Patients with Missing Maxillary Lateral Incisors. Journal of Clinical Orthodontics 2007; 41(9) 563-573.

[70] Thoraton L. Anterior Guidance: Group Function/Canine Guidance. A Literature Review. The Journal of Prosthetic Dentistry 1990; 64(4) 479-482.

[71] Huth KC, Nazet M, Paschos E, Linsenmann R, Hickel R, Nolte D. Autotransplantation and Surgical Uprighting of Impacted or Retained Teeth: A Retrospective Clinical

Study and Evaluation of Patient Satisfaction. Acta Odontologica Scandinavica 2013; 71(6) 1538–1546.

[72] Blomlof L, Lindskog S, Andersson L, Hedstrom KG, Hammarstrom L. Storage of Experimentally Avulsed Teeth In Milk Prior to Replantation. Journal of Dental Research 1983; 62(8) 912-916.

[73] Oswald RJ, Harrington GW, Van Hassel HJ. Replantation 1: The Role of the Socket. Journal of Endodontics 1980; 6(3) 479-484.

[74] Andersson L, Lindskog S, Blomlof L, Hedstrom KG, Hammarstrom L. Effect of Masticatory Stimulation on Dentoalveolar Ankylosis After Experimental Tooth Replantation. Endodontics Dental Traumatology 1985; 1(1) 13-6.

[75] Andreasen JO. The Effect of Pulp Extirpation or Root Canal Treatment on Periodontal Healing After Replantation of Permanent Incisors in Monkeys. Journal of Endodontics 1981; 7(6) 245-252.

[76] Gonnissen H, Politis C, Schepers S, Lambrichts I, Vrielinck L, Sun Y, et al. Long-Term Success and Survival Rates of Autogenously Transplanted Canines. Oral Surgery Oral Medicine Oral Pathology Oral Radiology and Endodontics 2010; 110(5) 570–578.

[77] Patel S, Fanshawe T, Bister D, Cobourne MT. Survival and Success of Maxillary Canine Autotransplantation: A Retrospective Investigation. European Journal of Orthodontics 2011; 33(3) 298–304.

[78] Hall GM, Reade PC. Root Resorption Associated with Autotransplanted Maxillary Canine Teeth. The British Journal of Oral Surgery 1983; 21(3) 179-191.

[79] Andreasen JO. Ectopic Eruption of Permanent Canines Eliciting Resorption of Incisors. Tandlaegebladet 1987; 91(11) 487-492.

[80] Shatz JP, Byloff F, Bernhard JP, Joho JP. Severely Impacted Canines: Autotransplantation as an Alternative. International Journal of Adult Orthodontics and Orthognathic Surgery 1992; 7(1) 45-52.

[81] Kristerson L. Autotransplantation of Human Premolars. International Journal of Oral Surgery 1985; 14(2) 200-213.

[82] Oshimi H. Nemawashi Jiggling and Gingival Muffler in Autogenous Tooth Transplantation. Nippon Dental Review 1993; 607: 65-74.

[83] Suzaki Y, Matsumoto Y, Kanno Z, Soma K. Preapplication of Orthodontic Forces to the Donor Teeth Affects Periodontal Healing of Transplanted Teeth. Angle Orthodontist 2008; 78(3) 495-501.

[84] Ru N, Bai Y. Canine Autotransplantation: Effect of Extraction Site Preservation with a Titanium Prosthesis and a Bioresorbable Membrane. American Journal of Orthodontics and Dentofacial Orthopedics 2013; 143(5) 724-734.

[85] Schatz JR, Joho JR. A Clinical and Radiographic Study of Autotransplanted Impacted Canines. International Journal of Oral and Maxillofacial Surgery 1993; 22(6) 342-346.

[86] Arikan F, Nizam N, Sonmez S. 5-Year Longitudinal Study of Survival Rate and Periodontal Parameter Changes at Sites of Maxillary Canine Autotransplantation. Journal of Periodontology 2008; 79(4) 595–602.

[87] Gonnissen H, Politis C, Schepers S, Lambrichts I, Vrielinck L, Sun Y, et al. Long-Term Success and Survival Rates of Autogenously Transplanted Canines. Oral Surgery Oral Medicine Oral Pathology Oral Radiology and Endodontics 2010; 110(5) 570–578

[88] Pogrel MA. Evaluation of Over 400 Autogenous Tooth Transplants. Journal of Oral and Maxillofacial Surgery 1987; 45(3) 205–211.

[89] Ahlberg K, Bystedt H, Eliasson S, Odenrick L. Long-Term Evaluation of Autotransplanted Maxillary Canines with Completed Root Formation. Acta Odontologica Scandinavica 1983; 41(1) 23–31.

[90] Zachrisson BU, Thilander B. Introduction to Orthodontics, 5th Edn. Stockholm: Tandlakaförlaget; 1985.

[91] Lewis PD. Preorthodontic Surgery in the Treatment of Impacted Canines. American Journal of Orthodontics 1971; 60(4) 383-397.

[92] Nordenvall KJ. Glass Ionomer Cement Used as Surgical Dressing After Radical Surgical Exposure of Impacted Teeth. Swedish Dental Journal 1992(3) 16: 87-92.

[93] Kohavi D, Becker A, Zilberman Y. Surgical Exposure, Orthodontic Movement, and Final Tooth Position as Factors in Periodontal Breakdown of Treated Palatally Impacted Canines. American Journal of Orthodontics 1984; 85(1) 72-77.

[94] Fournier A, Turcottej, Bernard C. Orthodontic Considerations in the Treatment of Maxillary Impacted Canines. American Journal of Orthodontics 1982; 81(3) 236-239.

[95] Stellzig A, Basdra EK, Kourposch G. The Etiology of Canine Tooth Impaction: A Space Analysis. Fortschritte Der Kieferorthopadie 1994; 55(3) 97-103.

[96] Vanarsdall RL Jr. Efficient Management of Unerupted Teeth: A Time-Tested Treatment Modality. Seminars in Orthodontics 2010; 16(3) 212-221.

[97] Becker A, Brin I, Ben-Bassat Y, Zilberman Y, Chaushu S. Closed-Eruption Surgical Technique for Impacted Maxillary Incisors: A Postorthodontic Periodontal Evaluation. American Journal of Orthodontics and Dentofacial Orthopedics 2002; 122(1) 9-14.

[98] Vermette M, Kokich V, Kennedy D. Uncovering Labially Impacted Teeth: Closed Eruption and Apically Positioned Flap Techniques. Angle Orthodontist 1995; 65(1) 23-32.

[99]   Vanarsdall R, Corn H. Soft Tissue Management of Labially Positioned Unerupted Teeth. American Journal of Orthodontics 1977; 72(1) 53-64.

[100] Kokich VG, Mathews DA. Impacted Teeth: Surgical and Orthodontic Considerations. In: JA McNamara Jr. (ed.) Orthodontics and Dentofacial Orthopedics. Ann Arbor, Michigan: Needham Press; 2001.

[101] Caprioglio A, Vanni A, Bolamperti L. Long-Term Periodontal Response to Orthodontic Treatment of Palatally Impacted Maxillary Canines. European Journal of Orthodontics 2013; 35(3) 323–328.

[102] Kuftinec MM, Stom D, Shapira Y. The Impacted Maxillary Canine: I. Review of Concepts. ASDS Journal of Dentistry for Children 1995; 62(5) 317-324.

[103] Tulcan T. An Evaluation of Treatment Outcomes of Labially Impacted Maxillary Canines. PhD Thesis, Department of Orthodontics, Philadelphia; 1997.

[104] Graber TM, Vanarsdall RL Jr. Orthodontics Current Principles and Techniques 3rd Ed. St Louis: Mosby; 2000.

[105] Schmidt A. Periodontal Reaction to Early Uncovering, Autonomous Eruption, and Orthodontic Alignment of Palatally Impacted Maxillary Canines. PhD Thesis. University of Washington, Seattle; 2004.

[106] Schmidt AD, Kokich VG. Periodontal Response to Early Uncovering, Autonomous Eruption, and Orthodontic Alignment of Palatally Impacted Maxillary Canines. American Journal of Orthodontics and Dentofacial Orthopedics 2007; 131(4) 449-455.

[107] Becker A, Shpack N, Shteyer A. Attachment Bonding to Impacted Teeth at the Time of Surgical Exposure. European Journal of Orthodontics 1996; 18(5) 457-463.

[108] Becker A. The Orthodontic Treatment of Impacted Teeth. Oxford, London: Wiley-Blackwell; 2012.

[109] Becker A, Chaushu S. Palatally Impacted Canines: The Case for Closed Surgical Exposure And Immediate Orthodontic Traction 2013; 143(4) 451-459.

[110] Burden DJ, Mullally BH, Robinson SN. Palatally Ectopic Canines: Closed Eruption Versus Open Eruption. American Journal of Orthodontics and Dentofacial Orthopedics 1999; 115(6) 640-644.

[111] Parkin NA, Milner RS, Deery C, Tinsley, Smith AM, Germain P, Freeman JV, Bell SJ, Benson PE. Periodontal Health of Palatally Displaced Canines Treated with Open Or Closed Surgical Technique: A Multicenter, Randomized Controlled Trial. American Journal of Orthodontics and Dentofacial Orthopedics 2013; 144(2) 176-184.

[112] Parkin N, Benson PE, Thind B, Shah A. Open Versus Closed Surgical Exposure of Canine Teeth That are Displaced in the Roof of the Mouth. The Cochrane Database of Systematic Reviews 2008; 8(4) CD006966

[113] Smailiene D, Kavaliauskiene A, Pacauskiene I, Zasciurinskiene E, Bjerklin K. Palatally Impacted Maxillary Canines: Choice of Surgical Orthodontic Treatment Method Does not Influence Post-Treatment Periodontal Status. A Controlled Prospective Study. European Journal Of Orthodontics 2013; 35(6) 803–810.

[114] Kuftinec MM, Shapiray. The Impacted Maxillary Canine: II. Surgical Consideration and Management. Quintessence International Dental Digest 1984; 15(9): 895-897.

[115] Sinha PK, Nanda RS. Management of Impacted Maxillary Canines Using Mandibular Anchorage. American Journal of Orthodontics and Dentofacial Orthopedics 1999; 115(3) 254-257.

[116] Goodsell JF. Surgical Exposure And Orthodontic Guidance of the Impacted Tooth. Dental Clinics of North America 1979; 23(3) 385–392.

[117] Mclaughlin R, Bennett C, Trevisi HJ. Systemized Orthodontic Treatment Mechanics 1st Ed. Barcelona, Spain: Mosby; 2002.

[118] Crescini A, Clauser C, Giorgetti R, Cortelini P, Pini Prato GP. Tunnel Traction of İnfra-Osseous Maxillary Canines: A Three Year Periodontal Follow-Up. American Journal of Orthodontics and Dentofacial Orthopedics 1994; 105(1) 61-72.

[119] Shapira Y, Kuftinec MM. Treatment of Impacted Cuspids the Hazard Lasso. Angle Orthodontist 1981 ; 51(3) 203-207.

[120] Celi D, Catalfamo L, Deli R. Palatally Impacted Canines:The Double Traction Technique. Progress in Orthodontics 2007; 8(1) 16-26.

[121] Bowman SJ, Carano A. The Kilroy Spring for Impacted Teeth. Journal of Clinical Orthodontics 2003; 37(12) 683-688.

[122] Shastri D, Nagar A, Tandon P. Alignment of Palatally Impacted Canine with Open Window Technique and Modified K-9 Spring. Contemporary Clinical Dentistry 2014; 5(2) 272–274.

[123] Vardimon AD, Graber TM, Drescher D, Bourauel C. Rare Earth Magnets and Impaction. American Journal of Orthodontics and Dentofacial Orthopedics 1991; 100(6) 494-512.

[124] Mcdonald E Yap WL. The Surgical Exposure and Application of Direct Traction of Unerupted Teeth. American Jounal of Orthodontics 1982; 89(4) 331-340.

[125] Kocsis A, Seres L. Orthodontic Screws to Extrude Impacted Maxillary Canines. Journal of Orofacial Orthopedics 2011; 73(1) 19-27.

[126] Poggio PM, Incorvati C, Velo S, Carano A. "Safe Zones": A Guide for Miniscrew Positioning in the Maxillary and Mandibular Arch. Angle Orthodontist 2006; 76(2)191–197.

[127] Chaushu S, Chaushu G. Skeletal Implant Anchorage in the Treatment of Impacted Teeth—A Review of the State of the Art. Seminars in Orthodontics 2010; 16: 234-241.

[128] Becker A, Kohavi D, Zilberman. Periodontal Status Following the Alignment of Palatally Impacted Canine Teeth. American Journal of Orthodontics 1983; 84(4) 332-336.

[129] Woloshyn H, Årtun J, Kennedy DB, Joondeph DR. Pulpal and Periodontal Reactions to Orthodontic Alignment of Palatally Impacted Canines. Angle Orthodontist 1994; 64(4) 257-264.

[130] Clark D. The Management of Impacted Canines: Free Physiologic Eruption. Journal of the American Dental Association 1971; 82(4) 836-840.

[131] D'Amico RM, Bjerklin K, Kurol J, Falahat B. Long-Term Results of Orthodontic Treatment of Impacted Maxillary Canines. Angle Orthodontist 2003; 73(3) 231-238.

[132] Becker A, Chaushu G, Chaushu S. Analysis of Failure in the Treatment of Impacted Maxillary Canines. American Journal of Orthodontics and Dentofacial Orthopedics 2010; 137(6) 743-754.

[133] Becker A, Chaushu S. Success Rate and Duration of Orthodontic Treatment for Adult Patients with Palatally Impacted Canines. American Journal of Orthodontics and Dentofacial Orthopedics 2003; 124(5) 509–514.

[134] Haney E, Gansky SA, Lee JS, Johnson E, Maki K, Miller AJ, Huang JC. Comparative Analysis of Traditional Radiographs and Cone-Beam Computed Tomography Volumetric Images in the Diagnosis and Treatment Planning of Maxillary Impacted Canines. American Journal of Orthodontics and Dentofacial Orthopedics 2010; 137(5) 590-597.

[135] Koutzoglou SI Kostaki A. Effect of Surgical Exposure Technique, Age, and Grade of Impaction on Ankylosis of an Impacted Canine, and the Effect of Rapid Palatal Expansion on Eruption: A Prospective Clinical Study. American Journal of Orthodontics and Dentofacial Orthopedics 2013; 143(3) 342-352.

[136] Pithon MM, Bernardes LA. Treatment of Ankylosis of the Mandibular First Molar with Orthodontic Traction Immediately After Surgical Luxation. American Journal of Orthodontics and Dentofacial Orthopedics 2011; 140(3) 396-403.

[137] Turley PK, Crawford LB, Carrington KW. Traumatically Intruded Teeth. Angle Orthodontist 1987; 57(3) 234-244.

[138] Puricelli E. Treatment of Retained Canines by Apicotomy. RGO 1987; 35(4) 326-330.

[139] Puricelli E. Apicotomy: A Root Apical Fracture for Surgical Treatment of Impacted Upper Canines. Head Face Med 2007; 6(3) 33.

[140] Becker A, Abramovitz I, Chaushu S. Failure of Treatment of Impacted Canines Associated with Invasive Cervical Root Resorption. Angle Orthodontist 2013; 83(5) 870-876.

5

Epithelial-Mesenchymal Transition — A Possible Pathogenic Pathway of Fibrotic Gingival Overgrowth

Ileana Monica Baniță, Cristina Munteanu,
Anca Berbecaru-Iovan, Camelia Elena Stănciulescu,
Ana Marina Andrei and Cătălina Gabriela Pisoschi

1. Introduction

Gingival overgrowth (GO) or gingival enlargement refers to important changes of gums aspect and function. Even it seems an issue of little significance, health of gums is a prerequisite condition for a psychological and physical comfort because severe GO affects speech, mastication, and nutrition, causes aesthetic concerns and increases susceptibility for periodontal and systemic diseases. The treatment of severe cases needs gingivectomy that may be repeated if is necessary.

At clinical endo-oral examination, GO is characterized by increased gums volume, swollen and deepening of gingival sulcus. Thickening of soft tissues covering alveolar ridges is more than 1 mm comprising both the mobile and attached gums. The degree of overgrowth can be variable from the interdentally papilla to cover the entire tooth crown. Enlargement is painless, slowly progressive and depends to a great extend on the oral hygiene [1-6].

Usually, GO is classified according the clinical appearance and the etiological factor. Histological and cell molecular studies have uncovered some of the pathogenic pathways and cellular alterations associated with GO but still remain unknown aspects.

In this chapter we describe recent insights into the pathogenic mechanisms of GO overgrowth discussing in detail the role of epithelial-mesenchymal transition (EMT) in gingival fibrotic diseases.

2. Terms definition, classification and risk factors for gingival overgrowth

Gingival overgrowth (GO), often named gingival hyperplasia or hypertrophy, is classified according the clinical appearance and the etiological factors, if these are known. If clinical examination displays rather an inflammatory aspect (gingivitis and periodontitis) the gums are red, soft, shiny, and bleed easily. Inflammatory gingivitis is induced frequently by poor dental hygiene resulting in bacterial plaque and causes reactive GO, named also focal reactive GO, inflammatory hyperplasia or epulis. Generally, the epulides are pedunculated or sessile lesions of gums; because this term, considered unsuitable, is clinico-topographical, without a histological description of the lesion, nowadays the preferred term is gums reactive lesion [7, 8]. Smoking, systemic diseases (diabetes mellitus, HIV infection) determine also inflammatory gums lesions.

Non inflamed gingival enlargement tends to have a darker red or purple color, is either firm or soft, when bleeds easily. Determinative causes are extremely polymorphous: (i) subjects with poor dental hygiene; (ii) specific hormonal states-puberty, pregnancy; (iii) nutritional deficiency, such as scurvy; (iv) blood conditions, such as acute leukemia, lymphoma or aplastic anemia; (v) genetic conditions – epulis or Neumann tumor; (vi) drug-induced GO (named also fibrotic gingival hyperplasia) appeared after administration of some anticonvulsivants (phenytoin), immunosupressants (cyclosporin A, CsA) and antihypertensive calcium channel blockers (verapamil, diltiazem, nifedipine); (vii) systemic diseases such as sarcoidosis, Crohn disease, acromegaly, primary amyloidosis or type I neurofibromatosis [6,9,10].

Gingival fibromatosis (GF) is the term frequently used for any GO when suspect a hereditary pattern (hereditary gingival fibromatosis, HGF), as part of a more extensive syndrome (Table 1) or the etiologic factor remains unknown-idiopathic gingival fibromatosis (IGF). Specialty literature is sometimes confuse or redundant regarding the relation between definition and the etiological factors. For the beginning, we tried to present a brief synthesis of these definitions.

Hereditary gingival fibromatosis (HGF), previously known as gingival elephantiasis, idiopathic gingival fibromatosis, hereditary gingival hyperplasia, non-bacterial plaque gingival lesion, gingival gigantism or just hypertrophic gums [11,12] can be classified as follows:

i.   Hereditary or isolated GF named also non-syndromic or type I GF seems to be determined by the mutation of SOS1 (*Sun of sevenless-1*) gene on chromosome 2. For the first time, this mutation was described in a large Brazilian family [13]. SOS1 is an oncogene involved in cell growth. This mutation was designated GINGF1 (Mendelian Inheritance in Man classification MIM135300) [10].

Recently a type 2 HGF, GINGF2 (MIM605544), was described in association to a mutation mapped on chromosome 5 but the specific gene involved has not yet been identified [10,14-16]. The presence of teeth in alveoli seems to be a condition for hereditary GO development as it disappears or reduces after tooth extraction. Some authors consider HGF an atypical pathology of childhood because it is present mainly during the mixed dentition stage [11]. Another type of HGF with family aggregation, GINGF3 (MIM 609955), a mutation mapped on chromosome

2 but not to the SOS 1 gene in which clinical signs appear earlier during the primary dentition stage was described by [17].

ii.   Syndromic GF is associated with several clinical signs in some syndromes (Table 1). In syndromic GF, gingival events are caused by chromosomal abnormalities (duplications, deletions) of chromosomes 2p12-16 [18,19], 4q (MIM252500), 8 (MIM266270), 14q [20], 19p (MIM266200), 19q (MIM248500) and Xq [8,9,13,21-26].

Syndrome	Clinical signs
Zimmerman-Laband Syndrome	GF and facial deformability, changes of nose and ears, nail dystrophy, hypoplasia, epilepsy, hepato-splenomegaly, deafness, mental retardation
Rutherford Syndrome	GF and corneal dystrophy, aggressive behavior, mental retardation
Jones Syndrome	GF and progressive deafness, maxillary odontogenic cysts
Cross Syndrome	Gingival hypertrophy and microphthalmia, mental retardation, hypopigmentation
Murray-Puretic-Drescher Syndrome	GF and bone, cartilage, skin and muscle diseases
Ramon Syndrome	GF and cherubism, hypertrichosis, mental retardation, convulsions, growth retardation, juvenile rheumatoid arthritis
Cowden Syndrome	Localized GF with multiple hamartomas

Table 1. Syndromic gingival fibromatosis [adapted after 6,15,16,27]

Recently, in [28] is described a new syndrome that includes generalized thin *hypoplastic amelogenesis imperfecta* found in a family with multiple consanguineous marriages, this type having clinical and histological similarities with GINGF1 and GINGF3.

Genetic and syndromic fibromatosis are sometimes termed IGF [12,27,29-32].

Lacking specific immunohistochemical markers, the diagnosis of HGF is based exclusively on clinical examination, patient medical history and family pedigree.

It was recommended to use the term „idiopathic fibromatosis" only for GF that doesn't incriminate genetic and hereditary causes mentioned above, in order to avoid these confusions of classification [6,9].

GO incidence varies according the socioeconomic status and the risk factors involved being reported a rate of 1/9000 adults; the most numerous GO are inflammatory or induced by drugs-phenytoin increases gingival volume in 57% of cases, CsA in 30-46% and calcium channel blockers in 10% [3,33,34]. HGF is the most rare type of GO and estimated to affect 1/750,000 people with the same incidence in both sexes [2,6,10,35,36].

Under the influence of such risk factors, clinical increase of gums volume is due to the enlargement of both epithelial and connective tissue. Microscopically examination displays the coexistence of tissue hypertrophy and cellular hyperplasia which imposed the generic term of GO [2]. Irrespective the risk factor, presence of bacterial plaque and hereditary predisposition are constantly incriminated as etiological cofactors mainly for drug-induced GO [2]. To sustain this association, it was revealed that patients with inflammatory GO before the onset of treatment with CsA developed more severe forms of GO [37] and suggested that patients carriers of a genetic polymorphism related to IL-1A expression often develop GO after CsA treatment [38]; specialty literature reports cases of IGF or HGF associated with chronic or aggressive periodontitis [39-41].

3. Histological aspects of gingival fibromatosis

Histological studies that we performed on samples of fibrotic gingival tissues revealed common, non-specific aspects despite the numerous risk factors, generally characterized by an increase of gums volume to which contribute both the epithelium (cellular hyperplasia) and lamina propria (accumulation of extracellular matrix, ECM, and cells) (Figure 1). Various types of GF are characterized by different incidence of pro-inflammatory cells.

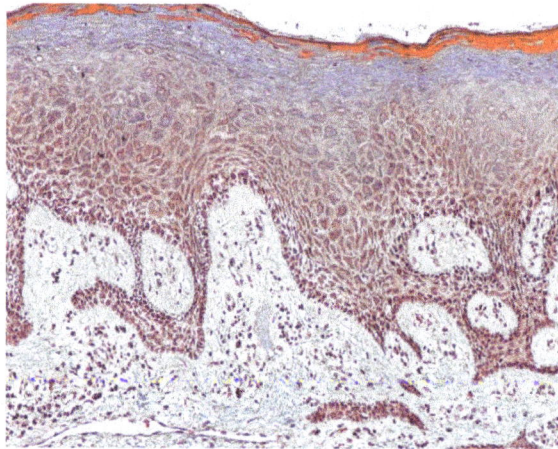

Figure 1. General view of a sample with gingival overgrowth (trichrome staining, x100)

In drug-induced GO, connective tissue is more rich in pro-inflammatory cells than in HGF or IGF. An exception is phenytoin-induced GO characterized mainly by fibrotic lesions unlike CsA or nifedipine-induced GO which determine important inflammatory reactions [23,42-45]. Due to its clinical and histological features, phenytoin-induced GO is often included in the category of fibromatous GO [11,15,23] which yield some confusions.

Histological changes of syndromic GO, HGF and phenytoin-induced GO are similar: epithelial hyperplasia with hyperkeratosis and elongated papillae, thickening of collagen bundles, increase of tissue differentiation and fluctuating number of fibroblasts (Figure 2a).

Enlargement and acanthosis of gingival epithelium with deep epithelial ridges was reported [46, 47]. Epithelial hyperplasia results from acanthosis but appears only in the areas of chronic inflammation [46-48]. In many areas epithelial hyperkeratosis was observed [17,26,47,49]. Regarding the sulcular epithelium we noted many signs of considerable degeneration, subpepithelial edema and extensive inflammatory cell infiltration (Figure 2b). Thick, densely wrapped collagen bundles with scattered resident cells of connective tissue were observed in lamina propria.

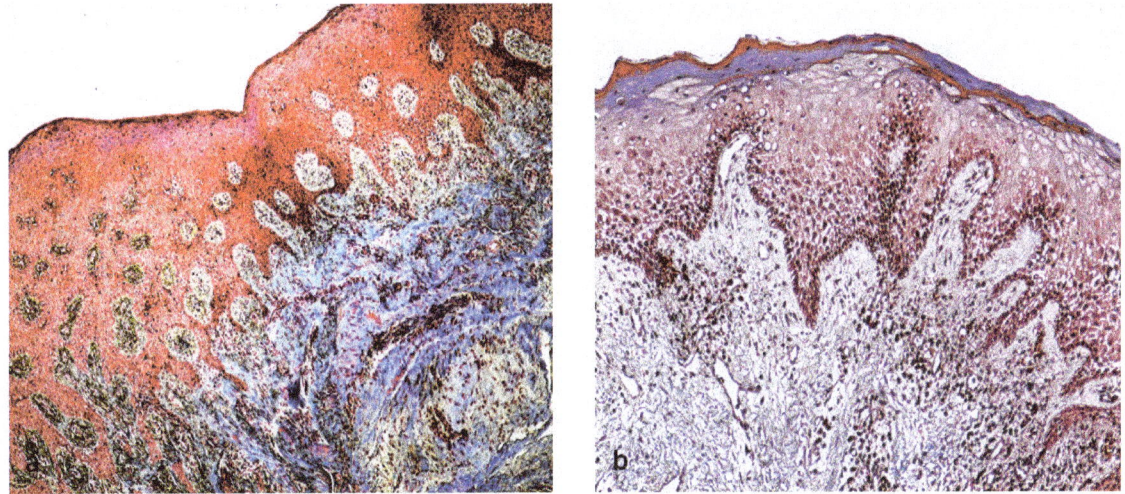

Figure 2. General view of syndromic GO: a) masticatory gingival mucosa; b) sulcular gingival mucosa (trichrome staining, x100)

The incidence of fibroblast is disputed; some authors reported numerous fibroblasts [16,31,45,50,51] while others claimed on the contrary a decreased number [17,41,43,52]. This variable number of fibroblasts even within HGF pointed attention to the different molecular mechanism underlying gingival fibrotic processes.

4. Pathogenic pathways of gingival overgrowth

Histological and cell molecular studies have uncovered some of the pathogenic pathways and cellular alterations associated with GO but still remain unknown aspects.

Studies revealed that the same molecules and biological events are involved in inflammation, wound repair and fibrosis. Theories and previous investigations on the morphology and molecular mechanisms by which the fibrotic deposition occurs have been widely published. Integrating these findings, Bartold and Narayanan state in [53] that fibrosis can evolve as a response to the action of a single factor or of a combination of various factors such as: (i) abnormal release of inflammatory mediators; synthesis of some molecules frees others and their crosstalk could have synergic, cumulative or antagonist effects; (ii) persistence of abnormal changes in the action of growth factors and cytokines; even the intensity of cell response to this stimulation is not so great the long lasting effect is cumulative and increased;

(iii) establishment of a pro-fibrotic cell phenotype; aberrant interaction of normal cell phenotypes with peptide mediators could induce the recruitment of abnormal cells.

These cell interactions determine the accumulation of gingival tissue through two main pathogenic pathways: (i) excessive synthesis of ECM and (ii) decrease of its breakdown [15,23,43,53-55]. Each of these pathways is initiated and sustained by growth factors, cytokines, molecules involved in ECM breakdown, matrix metalloproteinases – MMP, and their tissue inhibitors (TIMP) released by cellular elements that belongs both to the epithelium and gingival chorion. Recently, epithelial to mesenchymal transition (EMT) has been proposed as another pathogenic pathway promoting gingival fibrosis.

5. Role of epithelium in extracellular matrix accumulation — The epithelial-mesenchymal transition

Development of fibrotic lesions is indirectly related to the presence and histophysiology of epithelial cells. The interference of oral epithelial cells in ECM storage is sustained by the results of many studies reporting epithelial morphological changes besides the accumulation of connective tissue. In the same time, epithelial keratinocytes or inflammatory cells infiltrating the epithelium synthesize several biomolecules (growth factors, cytokines, MMPs and TIMPs) which alter collagen metabolism and ECM synthesis in the lamina propria. In a recent study, Menga and coworkers in [56] showed an intense expression of type 1 collagen and TIMP-1 in fibroblasts from mixed cultures of keratinocytes and fibroblasts obtained from patients with GF, in parallel to an increased rough endoplasmic reticulum. The authors suggested that keratinocytes play an important role in the pathogenesis of GF through increase of ECM storage. The epithelium suffers acanthosis and hyperkeratosis, increases the number of epithelial cells, and of many inflammatory cells infiltrating its deep layers. The increase of keratinocytes number determines not only the epithelial enlargement mainly in the spindle layer but also the appearance of many epithelial ridges ascending deep in the lamina propria. These epithelial ridges often branch and adhere one to another (Figure 1, and 2a, b).

These findings are constantly accompanied by the increase of keratinocyte mitotic activity proved by Ki-67 or PCNA immunostaining in [45,57-60]. In a recent study, using immunohistochemistry, [61] reported that Mcm-2 and Mcm-5 (members of minichromosome maintenance protein family), considered a novel class of proliferation markers, and geminin, also a proliferation marker according to [62], showed various expression in samples from three different families with GF. No differences between the expression of apoptotic markers Bcl-2 and Bax were observed among the group. Thus the authors concluded that an important heterogeneity of gingival fibrosis occurs. Epithelial cells proliferation is stimulated by pro-inflammatory cytokines and growth factors, such as KGF (Keratinocyte Growth Factor) or EGF (Epidermal Growth Factor). EGF and its receptors (EGfr) are positively correlated with the proliferative potential of the cells from rete pegs [63,64]. In a previous study, we observed that epithelial cells have an increased mitotic index in cases of GF highly infiltrated with inflammatory cells (Figure 3) (*unpublished data*).

Epithelial proliferation seems to have at least two functions in GO. First it ensure a continuous regeneration of keratinocytes, the regenerative capacity of the epithelium being compulsory when continuous desquamation of the superficial cells prevents bacterial colonization of the mucosa; second, epithelial proliferation could contribute to fibrosis by maintaining a cell pool to replace those cells involved in EMT and transformed in fibroblasts.

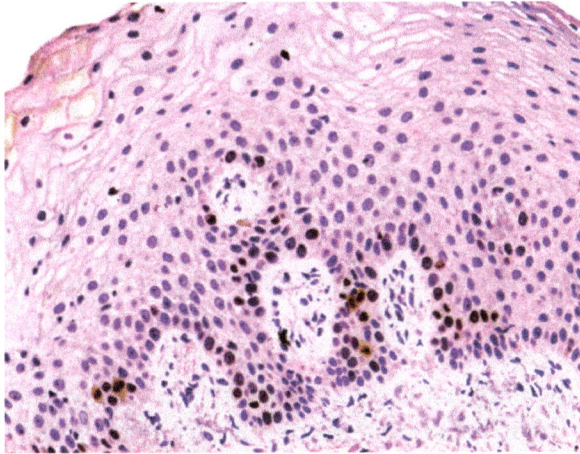

Figure 3. Gingival fibrosis. Increased number of Ki-67 positive cells in the basal epithelial layer (IHC, x200)

5.1. Concept of epithelial-mesenchymal transition

Epithelial-mesenchymal transition (EMT) is a concept first defined "epithelial–mesenchymal transformation" by G. Greenburg and E. Hay to characterize the conversion of epithelial cells to mesenchyme (EMT) and vice versa (mesenchymal-epithelial transition, MET) during chick embryonic development. This well-defined concept refers to a form of inherent plasticity of the epithelial phenotype that occurs normally in the developmental process. During EMT cells undergo a switch from a uniform, polarized epithelial phenotype to a motile mesenchymal phenotype. Current interest in this process stems from its importance in embryonic development and involvement in several pathologies (wound healing, fibrosis, cancer progression and metastasis) and has been extensively reviewed over the last 10 years in [65-78]. The conversion of an epithelial cell to a mesenchymal cell is critical to metazoan embryogenesis and a defining structural feature of organ development, and follows a common and conserved program with hallmarks [69,77]. As Lamouille and coworkers suggest in [77] it also has some variation which depend on the cell type, tissue environment and signals that activate the EMT program. During EMT, epithelial cell–cell and cell–ECM interactions are weakened and epithelial cells become able to trans-differentiate into fibrogenic fibroblast-like cells [68]. Turning an epithelial cell into a mesenchymal cell requires alterations in morphology, cellular architecture, adhesion, and migration capacity [69]. Loss of epithelial apical-basal polarity, acquisition of a front-rear polarity and motility result from the disappearance of cell adhesion molecules, reorganization of cytoskeleton and changes in cell shape [70]. In many cases cells gain an increased ability to break ECM proteins, acquire resistance to senescence and apoptosis [73].

Research in this field revealed that cellular events of EMT occurs in three distinct biological settings with different functional consequences: (i) type 1 EMT acts during implantation, embryogenesis and organ development when can generate mesenchymal cells (primary mesenchyme) and then secondary epithelia after the mesenchyme undergoes a reverse MET; (ii) type 2 EMT as a source of fibroblasts and other related cells involved in tissue regeneration and organ fibrosis in response to persistent inflammation; (iii) type 3 EMT occurs in neoplastic cells that have undergone genetic and epigenetic changes, notably of oncogenes and tumor suppressor genes, and contributes to cancer progression and metastasis [72,76,79]. A main distinction between the first two types of EMT is that type 1 EMT produces mesenchymal cells, whereas type 2 EMT results in fibroblasts in mature tissues. But other than the fact that mesenchymal cells have a shape similar to fibroblasts and, like fibroblasts, express fibronectin and fibrilar collagens, there is no evidence that fibroblasts originate in primitive mesenchymal cells [78].

EMT induction. Successful EMT depends upon a combination of growth factors and cytokines associated with the proteolytic digestion of the epithelial basement membranes (BM) under the action of MMPs. Local expression of TGF-β, EGF, IGF-II or FGF-2 facilitates EMT by binding membrane receptors with kinase activity [65]. The effect of TGF-β on EMT induction depends on β1-integrin transduction, Smad-dependent transcription, Smad-independent p38MAP kinase activation and Rho-like GTPase-mediated signaling [80,81]. IGF-II also facilitates the intracellular degradation of E-cadherin [82], while FGF-2 and TGF-β are required for the expression of MMP-2 and MMP-9 to assist in BM breakdown [83]. Indeed, decrease of type IV collagen from the BM was associated with increased expression of MMP-2 and MMP-9 during human pathologies involving EMT [54,84]. Loss of BM integrity is essential for the increased interactions between epithelial and connective tissue layers that contribute to fibrosis. Several lines of evidence indicate that TGF-β signaling is causally linked with EMT, plays an important role in regulating epithelial plasticity and is one of the most significant lines of communication between stroma and epithelium in different organ fibrosis (renal, cardiac, pulmonary, and hepatic) [81].

Consequent cell and molecular events are engaged to initiate EMT and enable it to complete: i) activation of transcription factors; ii) expression of cell surface specific proteins; iii) reorganization and expression of cytoskeletal proteins; iv) synthesis of ECM-degrading enzymes. In many cases, these factors are used as biomarkers to prove cell passage from one phenotype to the other and EMT involvement in tissue remodeling (Figure 4).

Transcriptional regulation of EMT. EMT involves changes in gene expression that induce the loss of proteins associated with the epithelial phenotype and increased expression of proteins associated with a mesenchymal and migratory cell phenotype with concomitant alterations in cytoskeletal organization, cell adhesion and production of ECM [72]. Cellular plasticity that is the switch of epithelial to mesenchymal features is achieved through a well orchestrated program that involves the action of three families of transcription factors: Snail, ZEB (zinc-finger E-box-binding) and bHLH (basic helix-loop-helix). Expression of these factors is induced in response to TGF-β through different mechanisms and their function is finely regulated at transcriptional, translational and post-translational levels [77].

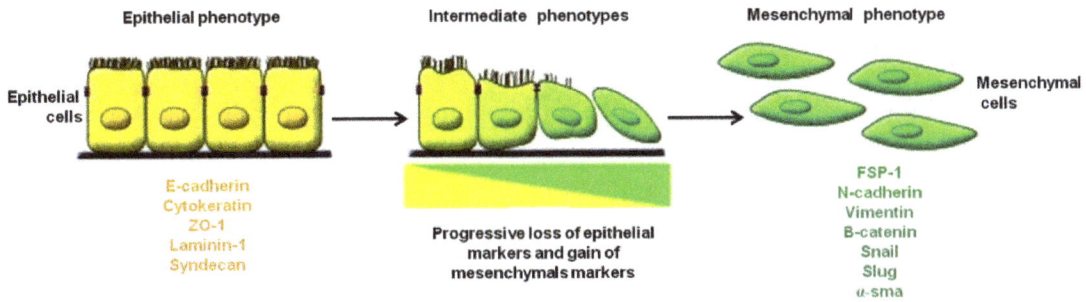

Figure 4. EMT is a functional transition from polarized epithelial cells into mobile cells able to secrete extracellular compounds (adapted after [72])

Snail family. Three Snail proteins have been identified in vertebrates: Snail 1 (Snail), Snail 2 (Slug) and Snail 3. They function as transcription repressors and their activity depend on the C-terminal zinc finger domain and the N-terminal SNAG domain [77]. Snail expression is induced in response to various growth factors. In cells that undergo TGF-β induced EMT Snail expression is mediated by Smad2/3 that form complexes with Smad4 and activates transcription by binding to Snail promoter [85]. Expression of Snails suppresses a spectrum of genes involved in maintaining the epithelial structure and function (Table 2) and enhances the expression of genes encoding vimentin and fibronectin leading to a full phenotype.

ZEB family. Two ZEB proteins have been identified in vertebrates, ZEB1 and ZEB2, which have two zinc-finger clusters at each end who mediates the interaction with DNA regulatory sequences. TGF-β induces the expression of ZEB proteins through an indirect mechanism mediated in part by Ets-1 and then ZEBs interact with Smad3 and repress the expression of epithelial marker genes (E-cadherin, claudins, ZO-3, plakophilin-2) and induce the expression of mesenchymal proteins (vimentin, N-cadherin, MMP-2) [86-88].

Helix-loop-helix family. HLH is a large family of transcription factors divided into seven classes based on their tissue distribution, dimerization ability and DNA-binding specificity [89]. The structure of HLH includes two parallel α-helices linked by a loop required for dimerization. E12, E47, Twist and Ids are involved in EMT. E12, E47 and Twist are able of DNA binding while Ids proteins are unable and act as dominant negative inhibitors [90]. Ectopic expression of E12 and E47 represses E-cadherin, plakoglobin or desmoplakin expression and induces mesenchymal markers, such as vimentin, fibronectin, N-cadherin or α5-integrin, and promotes migration and invasion [90]. Expression of Twist decreases E-cadherin, claudin-7 and occludin expression, increases that of N-cadherin and vimentin, and enhances migration and invasion [91]. Ids expression is repressed in response to TGF-β [92,93].

EMT proteome. Commonly used molecular markers of EMT could be grouped as follows: (i) decrease the amount of proteins associated with the epithelial phenotype; ii) abundance of some proteins; (iii) increased activity of selected proteins (Rho, GSK-3β); (iv) accumulation of proteins within the nucleus [69]. Table 2 listed common members of EMT proteome.

Delaminating of epithelia to facilitate movement is dependent on cell context and growth factor signaling and is accompanied by a decrease of apoptosis and mitosis [65].

In fibrotic diseases, TGF-β/Smad/Snail is a key signaling pathway [72,81]. Subsequently E-cadherin, cytokeratin, claudin and occludin are repressed, while FSP1 (fibroblast-specific protein-1), vimentin, fibronectin, Rho and MMP are increased [78].

According to [96] EMT represents the main source of fibroblasts in fibrotic pathology of connective tissues.

Generally, researches focused on few EMT markers and for this reason are not comprehensive. We specify that most information about the presence of EMT markers is indicated by the presence of proteins in epithelia and not only in fibroblasts, and as an example we'll discuss later the expression of FSP1.

	Name	EMT Type
Proteins that decrease in abundance	E-cadherin	1,2,3
	Cytokeratins	1,2,3
	Occludin	1,2,3
	Claudins	1,2,3
	ZO-1	1,2,3
	Collagen IV	1,2,3
	Laminin 1	1,2,3
Proteins that increase in abundance	N-cadherin	1,2
	Vimentin	1,2
	α-SMA	2,3
	Fibronectin	1,2
	FSP-1	1,2,3
	Snail, Slug	1,2,3
	ZEB	1,2,3
	Twist, E12/E47	1,2,3
	Ets-1	1,2,3
	MMP-2, MMP-9	2,3
	αvβ6 Integrin	1,3
Proteins that accumulate in the nucleus	β-catenin	1,2,3
	Smad2/3	1,2,3
	NF-κβ	2,3
	Snail, Slug	1,2,3
	Twist	1,2,3
	LEF-1	1,2,3
	Ets-1	1,2,3
	ZEB	1,2,3

Table 2. Epithelial-mesenchymal transition proteome (modified after [69,78])

FSP1, also known as S100A4 is one of the most interesting proteins identified in the EMT proteome [94]. This is a fibroblast-specific protein member of the S100 superfamily of cytoplasmic, calcium-binding proteins. S100 members have been implicated in calcium signal transduction, cytoskeletal membrane interactions, microtubule dynamics, p53-mediated cell cycle regulation, cellular growth and differentiation. Because the precise function of FSP1 is not entirely clear, its interaction with cytoskeletal moieties suggest that FSP1 protein may be associated with mesenchymal cell shape to enable motility and its expression indicates the presence of a molecular program determining the fibroblast phenotype in many organ fibrosis (kidney, liver, heart, brain, lungs) [72,94,95]. FSP1 is a specific marker not only for fibroblasts but also for endothelial cells undergoing endothelial-mesenchymal transition (EndMT) [78,96].

5.2. Epithelial-mesenchymal transition in gingival overgrowth

The process of EMT is involved in the normal development and several pathologies of oral cavity. In oral tissues, type 1 EMT is associated to palate and root development, type 2 EMT could play a contributory role in GF and oral submucous fibrosis and type 3 EMT is responsible for progression, invasion and poor prognosis of oral squamous cell carcinoma [76,97].

Fibrosis which occurs in many epithelial organs (kidney, liver, lung, heart, intestine) begins as a part of a repair event, that normally generate fibroblasts by EMT mechanism in order to reconstruct tissues following inflammatory injury. It seems that in gingival fibrosis as in other organs, the main trigger for type 2 EMT is the cytokine bath released in response to persistent inflammation [78,98]. Inflammatory injury results in the recruitment of a diverse array of cells (mainly resident fibroblasts and macrophages) that release growth factors (TGF-β, PDGF, EGF, FGF-2) and MMPs, especially MMP2, MMP3 and MMP 9 [72]. Under the influence of these factors and others chemoatractants [83] the delaminated epithelial cells migrate towards the disruptions of the BM. In EMT a discontinuous BM accompanied by a decreased expression of collagen IV and laminin was reported [54]. First the epithelial cells loss the polarity, cell adhesion molecules are disrupted and cell-cell junctions disappears. The intermediate filament profile change from cytokeratins to vimentin, the F-actin rearranges to a mesenchymal shape and some cells begin to express α-smooth muscle actin (α-sma) [83]. Epithelial cells undergoing EMT are specifically labeled *in vitro* and also *in vivo* [65,99,100] by FSP1, collagen type 1 and α-sma [78,94].

Recently, was provided data about EMT origin of gingival fibroblasts in drug-induced GO. The authors reported that mesenchymal cells from the lamina propria raised after phenotypic changes of some cells from the basal and parabasal epithelial layers [54,60, 101]. These cells had a diminished expression of E-cadherin compared to others; meanwhile the majority of keratinocytes expressed FSP1. Besides phenytoin-induced GO, we reported similarly results in a case of syndromic GO (Figure 5.) [47].

As we mentioned before, the main growth factor involved in EMT is TGF-β1 that triggers activation of the transcription factors able to repress the expression of epithelial markers, for example E-cadherin.

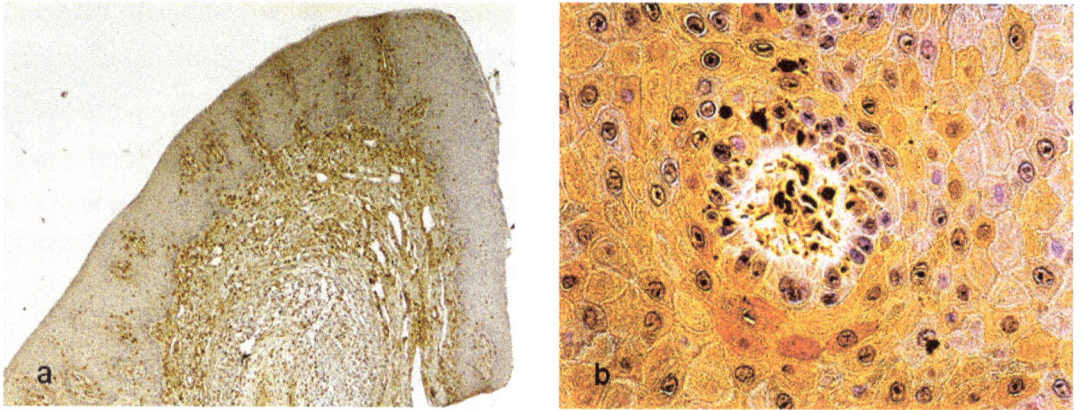

Figure 5. Syndromic GO. FSP1-positive reaction not only in fibroblasts but also in many keratinocytes, probably those that undergone EMT (IHC, a.x 100; b. x 400).

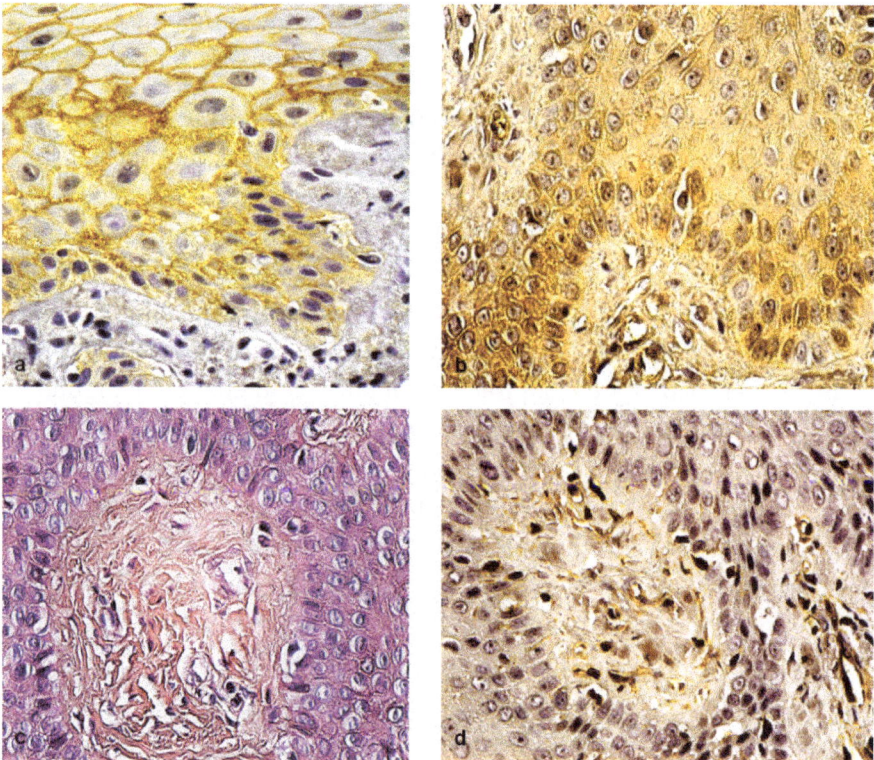

Figure 6. Idiopathic GO: a. Immunostaining for E-cadherin, x400; b. Immunostaining for TGF-β1, x200. c. Independent epithelial cells very close to the basal lamina, x400; d. FSP1 positive cells in the basal epithelium and the superficial connective tissue of the chorionic papilla, x 400.

Immunohistochemical studies that we performed on fibrotic GO samples revealed a diminished expression of E-cadherin in the basal epithelial layer in proximity of the BM suggesting that these cells undergo EMT while the immune reaction for TGF-β1 revealed many positive cells deep in the epithelium, mainly in the epithelial rete ridges [46,101]. A careful examination of these areas revealed independent epithelial cells detached from their neighbors, some of them extremely close to the basal lamina. In the lamina propria, adjacent to the BM we observed numerous intense FSP1 positive cells (Figure 6) (*unpublished data*).

The same results we reported in cases of phenytoin induced GO. Regarding the expression of FSP1 we observed an increased number of S100A4 positive cells both in the epithelium and lamina propria. At higher magnification we detected these FSP1 positive cells mainly in the basal epithelial layer nearby the disrupting BM and in the connective tissue close to the epithelium [101]. Tissues with phenytoin-induced GO showed significant reduction of E-cadherin expression in the epithelium compared with tissues from subjects without overgrowth where E-cadherin had a constant presence in the adherent junctions between keratinocytes. For the same samples we performed the assessment of the transcription factors Smad3 and Snail. We found an up-regulation in cells from profound epithelial layers. Often these positive cells were round or elongated, surrounded by a clear halo and we presumed that as a prove for lost of adhesion and the possibility to cross the disrupting BM to the connective tissue (Figure 7). Endothelial cells were also positive for these factors, especially for Smad3.

Overexpression of Snail, able to represses E-cadherin expression, and of MMP2 and MMP9 able to digest proteins from BM in the epithelium are downstream events of TGF-β1 biological effects [60, 102]. Experimental data proved that supplementation of epithelial cell cultures with TGF-β1 leads to loss of cell-cell adhesion through inhibition of E-cadherin gene expression and decrease of adherent junctions, tight junctions and desmosomes [72,102,103].

5.3. Connective tissue growth factor and the epithelial-mesechymal transition

As we mentioned before, besides TGF-β1 other growth factors could be involved in EMT such as IGF-II, EGF, FGF-2 and recently CTGF [104].

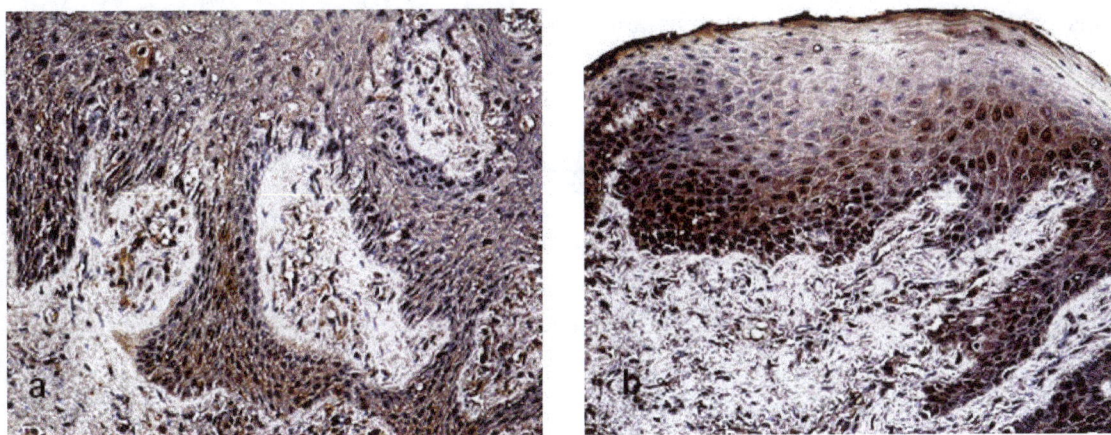

Figure 7. Phenytoin-induced GO. Expression of the transcription factors Smad 3 (a, x100) and Snail1 (b, x100).

TGF-β1 acts as a strong pro-fibrilogenetic factor through several mechanisms: (i) direct stimulation of collagen synthesis after the increase of number of highly collagen synthesizing fibroblasts through EMT; (ii) initiation of CTGF control on collagen synthesis [105]. Kantarci and coworkers in [104] showed a direct relation between the incidence of FSP1 positive cells and CTGF expression in drug-induced GO.

CTGF/CCN2 is a member of the CCN family whose members contain conserved cysteine-rich domains and have various biological activities, being important to stimulate proliferation of diverse cell types and to promote fibrosis [105]. CTGF/CCN2 is highly expressed in a wide variety of fibrotic lesions and was already demonstrated that CTGF levels are highest in gingival tissues from phenytoin induced lesions, intermediate in nifedipine-induced lesions, and nearly absent in CsA-induced overgrowth [44,106]. CTGF/CCN2 expression in connective tissue fibroblasts was positively related with the degree of fibrosis because CTGF is able to stimulate fibroblast proliferation and ECM synthesis.

We performed immunohistochemical studies to reveal the pattern of CTGF expression in various types of GO and we noted a constant intense CTGF positive reaction in all cases. We observed strong positivity in the epithelium and lamina propria not only in fibroblasts but also in endothelial and pro-inflammatory cells (Figure 8).

In phenytoin-induced GO and IGF, the most fibrotic types of GO, CTGF/CCN2 content was significantly higher compared to GO induced by other drugs (nifedipine, amlodipine) and controls. Similar results were reported by Kantarci and coworkers in [44] who revealed that CTGF/CCN levels were elevated in phenytoin-induced fibrotic lesions and HGF, the highest CTGF positive reaction being observed in the basal epithelial layer and the superficial connective tissue. Because the presence of CTGF in the epithelium is intriguing, they performed *in situ* hybridization to identify cells that express CTGF mRNA and confirmed the presence of a high amount of CTGF in the basal epithelial layer [44]. In the connective tissue, CTGF promotes local fibrosis but its presence in the epithelium could have a distinct significance as was mentioned for the uterine tissue where CTGF stimulates cell proliferation. The authors suggest that CTGF could also stimulate gingival cells proliferation, mesenchymal cells and also keratinocytes from the basal layer revealing an increased mitotic index in GO [44].

6. Role of mesenchymal cells in gingival overgrowth

The main cells of gingival connective tissue incriminated for increased collagen synthesis are logically the fibroblasts. Gingival fibroblasts are involved in ECM homeostasis through a dual effect. On the one hand, they are responsible for collagen synthesis and, on the other hand, by a process of phagocytosis, it performs ECM breakdown.

Under normal circumstances, but especially in organ fibrosis, fibroblasts show different origins. For example, in kidney fibrosis, the trans-differentiation of epithelial cells through EMT is responsible for 36% of fibroblasts, 14-15% originated in bone marrow stem cells-namely fibrocytes [99] and the rest from local fibroblast proliferation. [65]

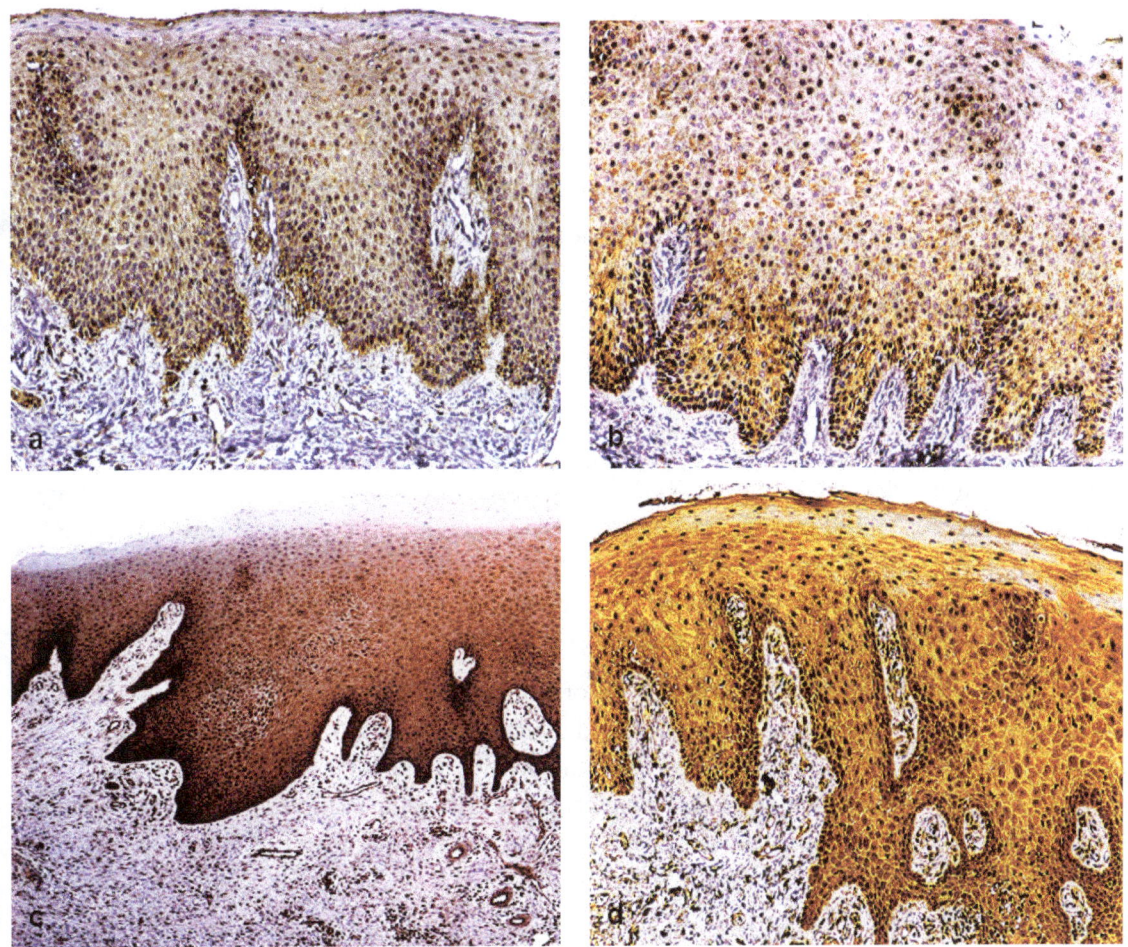

Figure 8. Immunostaining for CTGF in various samples of gingival fibromatosis: a, b. Idiopathic GF, x200, c. Phenytoin-induced GF, x100; d. Reactive GF, x200.

Kisseleva and Brenner showed in [99] that there are differences between the expression of several markers in fibrocytes and fibroblasts. The fibrocytes are cells involved in skin, kidney, liver and lung fibrosis. They have dual phenotypic features between fibroblasts and lymphocytes, and are defined as CD45+cells able to synthesize collagen with bone marrow origin, where they represents ≤1% of the cell population. Tissue injuries increase their number and after proliferation spread through blood into the damaged tissue where their proportion varies in relation to the tissue (5%-25%). [107,108]

In vitro the fibrocytes can differentiate into α-sma-positive myofibroblasts following stimulation by TGF-β1. The authors suggest that the role of these cells is not limited to tissue fibrilogenesis but to fulfill a role of intermediary in the biosignaling between the immune and fibrogenetic cells. This observation is based on the fact that fibrocytes express lymphoid markers (CD45, MHC II, MHC I), myeloid markers and adhesion molecules (CD54, ICAM-1) but also fibroblast markers (Thy-1, α-1 collagen). In addition, fibrocytes secrete growth factors and cytokines, for example TGF-β1, that stimulate the local deposition of ECM constituents. [109]

The second type of fibroblast-like cells derived still from bone marrow is represented by fibroblasts which in contrast to fibrocytes do not express myelo-monocytic markers and hyperexpress α-sma *in vitro* [110]. These are the main cells responsible for lung fibrosis.

Morphologically in fibrotic GO were described two populations of fibroblasts: one with little cytoplasm, considered inactive, and the other, well represented, with abundant cytoplasm, endoplasmic reticulum and Golgi apparatus-the active form. [29,111]

Kantarci and coworkers reported a reduction of fibroblasts apoptosis and at the same time an increased fibroblasts proliferation regardless of the inflammatory infiltration in phenytoin-induced GO and HGF which may explain the increased fibrosis. [45]

Through an autocrine signaling TGF-β1 seems to be the stimulus for increased collagen synthesis in fibroblasts. Hakkinen and Csiszar in [112] advanced the hypothesis that in GF the onset of overgrowth along with dental eruption can be placed either on account of the differentiation of abnormal phenotype fibroblasts or following their activation by pro-inflammatory cells or by mechanical trauma of eruption.

Recently there have been proposed two ways of stimulating fibroblasts proliferation either the pathway induced by increased FAS (fatty acid synthase) expression [112,113] or by increased expression of c-myc (a nuclear proto-oncogene) which hyperexpression is associated with disturbances of cell proliferation. [114] Conflicting results regarding the proliferative activity of fibroblasts in GF can be explained either by the genetic heterogeneity of the pathology itself or by the small number of cases studied. [112]

Cells that undergo EMT reorganize their actin cytoskeleton in order to facilitate formation of membrane projections that include sheet-like membrane protrusions or lamellipodia and spike-like extensions or filopodia that enable cells to directional motility. [115] Finally, the result of both EMT and EndMT is the myofibroblast, a mobile cell rich in actin stress fibers that expresses α-sma. These processes have been named EMyt and EndMyt. [77,116,117]. The mesenchymal phenotype resulting after EndMT is characterized by the acquisition of mesenchymal markers, such as α-sma and N-cadherin and the complementary loss of endothelial markers, such as CD31/Pecam-1 and VE-cadherin. [117] The mechanism of EndMT was discovered in the process of heart-development but actually it had been implicated in a wide variety of pathological conditions like several organs fibrosis and as well as in cancer. [98] There is not a consensus regarding the fact that myofibroblasts of fibrotic tissue occur exclusively as a result of EMT, these cells having a very heterogeneous origin. In tissue injury the local fibroblasts become activated by local cytokines released from inflammatory and resident cells or by the change of the mechanical microenvironment. These cells become first proto-myofibroblasts – cells acquiring contractile stress fibers composed of cytoplasmic actin. [118,119] *In vivo* such a protomyofibroblast became a differentiated myofibroblast by *de novo* expression of α-sma, used for this reason as a molecular marker. [119]

Since only certain subpopulations of myofibroblasts, previously called activated fibroblasts, express α-sma [120,121] it has advanced the hypothesis that actin of smooth muscle could actually label the cells detached from the blood vessel walls as a response to local injury. [122,123] At least three local events are needed to generate α-sma–positive differentiated myofibroblasts: (i). The accumulation of biologically active TGF-β1, the main promoter of fibroblasts differentiation into myofibroblasts and trigger of EMT; (ii) The presence of specialized ECM proteins, like the ED-A splice variant of fibronectin. Some authors argue that in the presence of the granulation tissue fibroblasts gain progressively features of myofibroblasts including α-sma expression [118,124] and (iii) High extracellular stress raised from the mechanical properties of ECM and cell remodeling activity. In addition, in [119] have been suggested that bone marrow derived circulating cells known as fibrocytes represent an alternative source of myofibroblasts in skin wound healing or organ fibrosis. There are few reports in the literature referring to the evidence of myofibroblasts in reactive focal GO, HGF and drug induced gingival hyperplasia. [25,47,126,127] Schor and coworkers reported in [128] that the only tissues that do not develop post lesion scars are embryonic and gingival tissues. This special reactivity was due to the fact that gingival fibroblasts and skin activates TGFβ1 by different signaling pathways. [129] Following the experiments authors suggested that the lack of scars in gingival mucosa is due to the fact that mechanical stress, a normal condition for functional periodontal tissues and remodeling processes is translated into fibroblast proliferation, production of TGF-β1 and CTGF, but not in activating genes responsible for α-sma synthesis.

7. Conclusions and perspectives

EMT is a dynamic physio-pathological event that depends upon a fine crosstalk between signaling pathways. Understanding the molecular mechanisms involved in EMT may reveal new biological targets for an effective therapeutic control of fibrosis in syndromic and IGF.

Further studies are needed regarding the expression of genes that control the synthesis of ECM under the particularities of structure and function of oral mucosa which normally is constantly remodeled and, on the other hand, is in a continuous state of inflammation due to the contact with different external agents. In this respect, special attention should be paid to factors that govern the relationship between innate immunity and EMT.

List of abbreviations

GO-Gingival Overgrowth

EMT – Epithelial-Mesenchymal Transition

GF-Gingival Fibromatosis

HGF-Hereditary Gingival Fibromatosis

IGF-Idiopathic Gingival Fibromatosis

IL1A – Interleukin 1A

ECM-Extracellular matrix

CsA-cyclosporin

MMP – Matrix Metalloproteinases

TIMP – Tissue Inhibitors of Matrix Metalloproteinases

KGF-Keratinocyte Growth Factor

EGF-Epidermal Growth Factor

EGFr – Epidermal Growth Factor receptor

MET – Mesenchymal Epithelial Transition

BM – Basement Membrane

TGF – Transforming Growth Factor

IGF – Insulin-like Growth Factor

FGF – Fibroblast Growth Factor

ZEB – Zinc finger E-box binding

bHLH – basic Helix-Loop-Helix

FSP1 – Fibroblast Specific Protein-1

EndMT – Endothelial Mesenchymal Transition

PDGF – Platelet Derived Growth Factor

α-sma-α-smooth muscle actin

CTGF – Connective Tissue Growth Factor

EMyt – Epithelial Myofibroblast Transition

EndMyt-Endothelial Myofibroblast Transition

Author details

Ileana Monica Baniță[1], Cristina Munteanu[1], Anca Berbecaru-Iovan[2],
Camelia Elena Stănciulescu[2], Ana Marina Andrei[2] and Cătălina Gabriela Pisoschi[2*]

*Address all correspondence to: c_pisoschi@yahoo.com

1 Department of Dentistry, University of Medicine and Pharmacy, Craiova, Romania

2 Department of Pharmacy, University of Medicine and Pharmacy, Craiova, Romania

References

[1] Desai P & Silver JG. Drug-induced gingival enlargements. Journal of Canadian Dental Association 1998;64(4):263-268

[2] American Academy of Periodontology. Informational paper: drug associated gingival enlargement. Journal of Periodontology 2004;75:1424-1431

[3] Kataoka M, Kido J, Shinohara Y & Nagata T. Drug-Induced Gingival Overgrowth-a Review. Biological and Pharmaceutical Bulletin 2005;28(10):1817-1821

[4] Lin K, Guihoto LMFF & Yacubian EMT. Drug-Induced Gingival Enlargement – Part II. Antiepileptic Drugs Not Only Phenitoin is Involved. Journal of Epilepsy and Clinical Neurophysiology 2007;13(2):83-88

[5] Carey JC, Cohen MM Jr, Curry CJ, Devriendt K, Holmes LB & Verloes A. Elements of morphology: standard terminology for the lips, mouth, and oral region. American Journal of Medical Genetic part A. 2009;149A(1):77-92.

[6] www.maxillofacialcenter.com

[7] Kfir Y, Buchner A & Hansen LS. Reactive lesions of the gingiva. A clinicopathological study of 741 cases. Journal of Periodontology 1980;51(11):655-661

[8] Savage NW & Daly CG. Gingival enlargements and localized gingival overgrowths. Australian Dental Journal 2010;55(Suppl 1):55-60

[9] Clocheret K, Dekeyser C, Carels C &, Willems G. Idiopathic gingival hyperplasia and orthodontic treatment case report. Journal of Orthodontics 2003;30(1):13-19

[10] http://dermnetnz.org.

[11] Bittencourt LP, Campos V, Moliterno LFM, Ribeiro DPB & Sampaio RK. Hereditary Gingival Fibromatosis Review of the Literature and a case report. Quintessence International 2000;31:415-418

[12] Coletta RD & Graner E. Hereditary gingival fibromatosis: a systematic review. Journal of Periodontology 2006;77(5):753-764

[13] Hart TC, Zhang Y, Gorry MC, Hart PS, Cooper M, Marazita ML, Marks JM, Cortelli JR & Pallos D. A mutation in the SOS1 gene causes hereditary gingival fibromatosis type1. The American Jounal of Human Genetics 2002;70(4):943-954

[14] Zhu Y, Zhang W, Huo Z, Zhang Y, Xia Y, Li B, Kong X & Hu L. A novel locus for maternally inherited human gingival fibromatosis at chromosome 11p15. Human Genetics 2007;121(1):113-123

[15] Douzgou S & Dallapicolla B. The gingival Fibromatoses, In: Underlying mechanisms of epilepsy, Kaneez FS (Editor), Intech, 2011, ISBN 978-953-307-765-9

[16] Ibrahim M, Abouzaid M, Mehrez M, Gamal El Din H. & El Kamah G. Genetic Disorders Associated with Gingival Enlargement, In: Gingival diseases – their aethiology,prevention and treatment. Panagos FD & Davies RB (Editors), Intech, 2011, ISBN 978-953-306-367-7

[17] Pampel M, Maier S, Kreczy A, Weirich-Schwaiger H, Utermann G & Janecke AR. Refinement of the GINGF3 locus for hereditary gingival fibromatosis. European Journal Pediatrics 2010;169(3):327-332

[18] Fryns JP. Gingival fibromatosis and partial duplication of the short arm of chromosome 2 (dup(2)(p13-p21). Annales de Genetique 1996;39(1):54-55

[19] Shashi V, Pallos D, Pettenati MJ, Cortelli JR, Fryns JP, von Kap-Herr C & Hart TC. Genetic heterogeneity of gingival fibromatosis on chromosome 2p. Journal of Medical Genetics 1999;36(9):683-686

[20] Rivera HM, Rramirez-Duenas L, Figuera LE, Gonzales-Montes RM & Vasquez AI. Opposite Inbalaces of distal 14q in two unrelated patients. Annales de Genetique 1992;35:97-100

[21] Marcias Flores MA, Garcia-Cruz D, Rovera H, Escobar-Lujan M, MelendezVeg A, Rivas-Campos D, Rodriguez-Colazzo F, Morello-Arellano I & Cantu JM. A new Form of Hipertrichosis inherited as an X-linked dominant trait. Human Genetics 1984:66(1):66-70

[22] Seymour RA, Ellis JS & Thomason JM. Risk factor for drug induced gingival overgrowth. Journal of Clinical Periodontology 2000;27:217-223

[23] Trackman PC & Kantarci A. Connective tissue metabolism and gingival overgrowth. Critical Review in Oral Biology and Medicine 2004; 15(3):165-175

[24] Taylor GW & Borgnakke WS. Periodontal disease: associations with diabetes, glycemic control and complications. Oral Disease 2008;14(3);191-203

[25] Damasceno LS., Gonçalves F da S, Costa e Silva E, Zenóbio EG, Souza PE & Horta MC. Stromal myofibroblasts in focal reactive overgrowths of the gingival. Brazilian Oral Research 2012;26(4):373-377

[26] Livada R & Shiloah J. Gummy smile: could it be genetic? Hereditary gingival fibromatosis. Journal of the Michigan Dental Association 2012;94(12):40-43

[27] Khan U, Mustafa S, Saleem Z & Azam A. Hereditary Gingival Fibromatosis, Diagnosis and treatment. Pakistan Oral & Dental Journal 2012;32(2):226-231

[28] Martelli-Júnior H, Bonan PR, Dos Santos LA, Santos SM, Cavalcanti MG & Coletta RD. Case reports of a new syndrome associating gingival fibromatosis and dental abnormalities in a consanguineous family. Journal of Periodontology 2008;79(7): 1287-1296

[29] DeAngelo S, Murphy J, Claman L, Kalmar J & Leblebicioglu B. Hereditary gingival fibromatosis: a review. Compendium of Continuing Education in Dentistry 2007;28(3):138-143

[30] Cekmez F, Pirgon O & Tanju IA. Idiopathic gingival hyperplasia. International Journal of Biomedical Sciences 2009;5(2):198-200

[31] Jaju PP, Desai A, Desai RS & Jaju SP. Idiopathic Gingival Fibromatosis: Case Report and Its Management. International Journal of Dentistry 2009, Vol.2009, Article ID 153603, 6 pages, doi:10.1155/2009/153603, ISSN 1687-8736

[32] Yadav VS, Chakraborty S, Tewari S & Sharma RK. An unusual case of idiopathic gingival fibromatosis. Contemporary Clinical Dentistry 2013;4(1):102-104

[33] Brunet L, Miranda J, Roset P, Berini L, Farre M & Mendieta C. Prevalence and risk of gingival enlargement in patients treated with anticonvulsant drugs. European Journal of Clinical Investigation 2001;31:781-788

[34] Seymour RA. Effects of medications on the periodontal tissues in health and disease. Periodontology 2000 2006;40:120-129

[35] Fletcher JP. Gingival Abnormalities of genetic origin: a preliminary communication with special reference to hereditary generalized gingival fibromatosis. Journal of Dental Research 1996;45:597-612

[36] Kather J, Salgado MA, Salgado UF, Cortelli JR & Pallos D. Clinical and histomorphometric characteristics of three different families with hereditary gingival fibromatosis. Oral Surgery Oral Medicine Oral Pathology Oral Radiology and Endodontology 2008;105(3):348-352

[37] Varga E, Lennon MA & Mair LH. Pre-transplant gingival hyperplasia predicts severe cyclosporin-induced gingival overgrowth in renal transplant patients. Journal of Clinical Periodontology 1998;25(3):225-230

[38] Bostanci N, Ilgenli T, Pirhan DC, Clarke FM, Marcenes W, Atilla G, Hughes FJ & McKay IJ. Relationship between IL-1A polymorphisms and gingival overgrowth in renal transplant recipients receiving cyclosporin A. Journal of Clinical Periodontology 2006;33(11):771-778

[39] Casavecchia P, Uzel MI, Kantarci A, Hasturk H, Dibart S, Hart TC, Trackman PC & Van Dyke T. Hereditary gingival fibromatosis associated with generalized aggressive periodontitis: a case report. Journal of Periodontology 2004;7(5):770-778

[40] Chaturvedi R. Idiopathic gingival fibromatosis associated with generalized aggressive periodontitis: a case report, Journal Canadian Dental Associattion 2009;75(4): 291-295

[41] Rizwan S. Gingival Fibromatosis with Chronic Periodontitis-A rare Case report. Inteernational e-Journal of Science, Medicine and Education 2009;3(2):24-27

[42] Uzel MI, Kantarci A, Hong HH, Uigur C, Sheff MC & Firatli E. Connective tissue growth factor in phenytoin induced gingival overgrowth. Journal of Periodontology 2001;72:921-931

[43] Uzel MI, Casavecchia P, Kantarci A, Gallagher G, Trackman PC & Van Dyke TE. 3000 Fibrosis Levels in Hereditary Gingival Fibromatosis, http//iadr.confex.com/iadr/2002 SanDiego

[44] Kantarci A, Black SA, Xydas CE, Murawel P, Uchida Y, Yucecal-Tuncer B, Atilla G, Emingil G, Uzel MI, Lee A, Firatli E, Sheff M, Hasturk H, Van Dyke TE, Trackman PC, Epithelial and Connective Tissue Cell CTGF/CCN Expression in Gingival Fibrosis, Journal of Pathology 2006; 210(1):59-66

[45] Kantarci A, Augustin P, Firatli E, Sheff MC, Hasturk H, Graves DT, Trackman PC., Apoptosis in gingival overgrowth tissues., Dental Research 2007;86(9):888-892

[46] Baniţă M, Pisoschi C, Stănciulescu C, Mercuţ V, Scrieciu M, Hâncu M & Crăiţoiu M. Phenytoin induced gingival overgrowth – an immunohistochemical study of TGF-β1 mediated pathogenic pathways. Farmacia 2011;59(1):24-34

[47] Pascu I, Pisoschi CG, Andrei AM, Munteanu C, Rauten AM, Scrieciu M, Taisescu O, Surpăţeanu M & Baniţă M. Heterogeneity of Collagen Secreting Cells in Gingival Fibrosis – an Immunohistochemical Assessment and a Review of the Literature. Romanian Journal of Morphology and Embryology (in press)

[48] Baniţă M, Pisoschi C, Stănciulescu C, Scrieciu M & Căruntu ID. Idiopathic gingival overgrowth – a morphological study an review of the literature. Revista Medico-Chirurgicală a Societăţii de Medici şi Naturalişti Iasi 2008;112(4):1076-1083

[49] Ramer M, Marrone J, Stahl B & Burakoff R. Hereditary gingival fibromatosis: identification, treatment, control. Journal of the American Dental Association 1996;127(4): 493-495

[50] Doufexi A, Mina M & Ioannidou E. Gingival overgrowth in children: epidemiology, pathogenesis, and complications. A literature review. Journal of Periodontology 2005;76(1):3-10

[51] Vishnoi SL. Hereditary Gingival Fibromatosis: Report of Four generations pedigree. International Journal of Case Reports and Images 2012;2(6):1-5.

[52] Tipton DA & Dabbous MK. Autocrine transforming growth factor beta stimulation of extracellular matrix production by fibroblasts from fibrotic human gingiva. Journal of Periodontology 1998; 69(6):609-619

[53] Bartold PM & Narayanan AS. Molecular and cell biology of healthy and diseased periodontal tissues. Periodontology 2000, 2006;40(1):29-49.

[54] Kantarci A, Nseir Z, Kim YS, Sume SS & Trackman PC. Loss of basement membrane integrity in human gingival overgrowth. Journal of Dental Research 2011;90(7): 887-893

[55] Aghili H & Goldani Moghadam M. Hereditary gingival fibromatosis: a review and a report of a rare case. Case Reports in Dentistry, Vol. 2013; Article ID:930972. doi: 10.1155/2013/930972

[56] Menga L, Yea X, Fan M, Xiong X, Von den Hoffb JW & Biana Z. Keratinocytes modify fibroblast metabolism in hereditary gingival fibromatosis. Archives of Oral Biology 2008;53(11):1050-1057

[57] Saito K, Mori S, Iwakura M & Sakamoto S. Immunohistochemical localization of transforming growth factor beta, basic fibroblast growth factor and heparan sulfate glycosaminoglycan in gingival hyperplasia induced by nifedipine and phenytoin. Journal of Periodontal Research 1996;31:545-555

[58] Ayanoglou CM & Lesty C. Cyclosporin A-induced gingival overgrowth in the rat: a histological, ultrastructural and histomorphometric evaluation. Journal of Periodontal Research 1999;34(1):7-15

[59] Martelli-Júnior H, Lemos DP, Silva CO, Graner E & Coletta RD. Hereditary gingival fibromatosis: report of a five-generation family using cellular proliferation analysis. Periodontology 2005;76(12):2299-2305

[60] Sume SS, Kantarci A, Lee A, Hasturk H & Trackman PC. Epithelial to mesenchymal transition in gingival overgrowth. The American Journal of Pathology 2010;177(1): 208-218

[61] Martelli-Júnior H, Santos C de O, Bonan PR, Moura P de F, Bitu CC, León JE & Coletta RD. Minichromosome maintenance 2 and 5 expressions are increased in the epithelium of hereditary gingival fibromatosis associated with dental abnormalities. Clinics (Sao Paulo) 2011;66(5):753-757

[62] Gonzales MA, Tachibana KE, Chin SF Callagy G, Madine MA, Vowler SL, Pinder SE, Laskey RA & Coleman N. Geminin predicts adverse clinical outcome in breast cancer by reflecting cell-cycle progression. Journal of Pathology 2004;204(2):121-130

[63] Araujo CS, Graner E, Almeida OP, Sauk JJ & Coletta RD. Histomorphometric characteristics and expression of epidermal growth factor and its receptor by epithelial cells of normal gingival and hereditary gingival fibromatosis. Journal of Periodontal Research 2003;38(3):237-241

[64] Bulut S, Uslu H, Ozdemir BH, Bulut OE, Analysis of proliferative activity in oral gingival epithelium in immunosuppressive medication induced gingival overgrowth, Head Face Medicine 2006; 2:13

[65] Kalluri R & Neilson E.G. Epithelial-mesenchymal transition and its implications for fibrosis. Journal of Clinical Investigation 2003;112(12):1776–1784

[66] Thiery JP. Epithelial mesenchimal transition in development and pathologies. Current Opinion in Cell Biology 2003;15(6):740–746

[67] Liu Y. Epithelial to mesenchymal transition in renal fibrogenesis: pathologic significance, molecular mechanism, and therapeutic intervention. Journal of the American Society of Nephrology 2004;15(1):1-12

[68] Radisky DC. Epithelial-mesenchymal transition. Journal of Cell Science 2005;118(19): 4325–4326

[69] Lee JM, Dedhar S, Kalluri R & Thompson EW. The epithelial-mesenchymal transition: new insights in signaling, development, and disease. Journal of Cell Biology 2006;172(7):973-981.

[70] Thiery JP & Sleeman JP. Complex networks orchestrate epithelial–mesenchymal transitions. Nature Reviews. Mollecular Cell Biology 2006;7(2):131–142

[71] Hugo H, Ackland ML, Blick T, Lawrence MG, Clements JA, Williams ED & Thompson EW. Epithelial--mesenchymal and mesenchymal--epithelial transitions in carcinoma progression. Journal of Cell Physiology 2007;213(2):374-383

[72] Kalluri R & Weinberg RA. The basics of epithelial-mesenchymal transition. Journal of Clinical Investigation 2009;119:1420–1428

[73] Thiery JP, Acloque H & Nieto MA. Epithelial-Mesenchymal Transitions in Development and Disease. Cell 2009;139: 871-890

[74] Cannito S, Novo E, Valfrè di Bonzo L, Busletta C, Colombatto S & Parola M. Epithelial–Mesenchymal Transition: From Molecular Mechanisms, Redox Regulation to Implications in Human Health and Disease. Antioxidant Redox Signaling 2010;12:1383-1430

[75] Carew RM, Wang B & Kantharidis P. The role of EMT in renal fibrosis. Cell Tissue Research 2012;347:103–116

[76] Ghanta SB, Nayan N, Raj Kumar NG & Pasupuleti S. Epithelial–mesenchymal transition: Understanding the basic concept. Journal of Orofacial Sciences 2012;4(2): 82-86

[77] Lamouille S, Xu J & Derynck R. Molecular mechanisms of epithelial-mesenchymal transition. Nature Reviews. Molecular Cell Biology 2014;15(3):178-196

[78] Zeisberg M & Neilson EG. Biomarkers for epithelial-mesenchymal transitions. The Journal of Clinical Investigation 2009;119(6):1429–1437

[79] Kalluri R. EMT:when epithelial cells decide to become mesenchymal-like cells. The Journal of Clinical Investigation 2009;119(6):1417-1419

[80] Bhowmick NA, Zent R, Ghiassi M, McDonnell M & Moses HL. Integrin beta 1 signaling is necessary for transforming growth factor-beta activation of p38MAPK and epithelial plasticity. The Journal of Biological Chemistry 2001;276(50):46707-46713

[81] Xu J, Lamouille S & Derynck R. TGF-β-induced epithelial to mesenchymal transition. Cell Research 2009;19:156-172

[82] Morali OG, Delmas V, Moore R, Jeanney C, Thiery JP & Larue L. IGF-II induces rapid beta-catenin relocation to the nucleus during epithelium to mesenchyme transition. Oncogene 2001;20(36):4942-4950

[83] Strutz F, Zeisberg M, Ziyadeh FN, Yang CQ, Kalluri R, Müller GA & Neilson EG. Role of basic fibroblast growth factor-2 in epithelial-mesenchymal transformation. Kidney International 2002;61(5):1714-1728

[84] Zeng ZS, Cohen AM & Guillem JG. Loss of basement membrane type IV collagen is associated with increased expression of metalloproteinases 2 and 9 (MMP-2 and MMP-9) during human colorectal tumorigenesis. Carcinogenesis 1999;20(5):749-755.

[85] Cho HJ, Baek KE, Saika S, Jeong MJ & Yoo J. Snail is required for transforming growth factor-beta-induced epithelial-mesenchymal transition by activating PI3 kinase/Akt signal pathway. Biochemical and Biophysical Research Communication 2007;353(2):337-343

[86] Postigo AA. Opposing functions of ZEB proteins in the regulation of the TGFb/BMP signaling pathway. EMBO Journal 2003;22 (10):2443-2452

[87] Vandewalle C, Comijn J, De Craene B, Vermassen P, Bruynee E., Andersen H, Tulchinsky E, van Roy F & Berx G. SIP1/ZEB2 induces EMT by repressing genes of different epithelial cell-cell junctions. Nucleic Acids Research 2005; 33(20):6566-6578

[88] Bindels S, Mestdagt M, Vandewalle C, Jacobs, N, Volders L, Noel A, van Roy F, Berx G, Foidart JM & Gilles C. Regulation of vimentin by SIP1 in human epithelial breast tumor cells. Oncogene 2006; 25(36):4975-4985

[89] Massari ME & Murre C. Helix-loop-helix proteins: regulators of transcription in eucaryotic organisms. Molecular Cell Biology 2000;20:429-440

[90] Perez-Moreno MA, Locascio A, Rodrigo I, Dhondt G, Portillo F, Nieto MA & Cano A. A new role for E12/E47 in the repression of E-cadherin expression and epithelial-mesenchymal transitions. The Journal of Biological Chemistry 2001;276(29): 27424-27431

[91] Ansieau S, Bastid J, Doreau A, Morel AP, Bouchet BP, Thomas C, Fauvet F, Puisieux I, Doglioni C, Piccinin S, Maestro R, Voeltzel T, Selmi A, Valsesia-Wittmann S, Caron de Fromentel C & Puisieux A. Induction of EMT by twist proteins as a collateral effect of tumor-promoting inactivation of premature senescence. Cancer Cell 2008;14(1):79-89

[92] Kang Y, Chen CR & Massagué J. A self-enabling TGFb response coupled to stress signaling: Smad engages stress response factor ATF3 for Id1 repression in epithelial cells. Molecular Cell 2003;11(4):915-926

[93] Kowanetz M, Valcourt U, Bergstrom R, Heldin CH & Moustakas A. Id2 and Id3 define the potency of cell proliferation and differentiation responses to transforming growth factor beta and bone morphogenetic protein. Molecular Cell Biology 2004;24(10):4241-4254

[94] Strutz F, Okada H, Lo CW, Danoff T, Carone RL, Tomaszewski JE & Neilson EG. Identification and characterization of a fibroblast marker: FSP1. The Journal of Cell Biology 1995;130(2):393-405

[95] Schneider RK, Neuss S, Stainforth R, Laddach N, Bovi M, Knuechel R & Perez-Bouza A. Three-dimensional epidermis-like growth of human mesenchymal stem cells on dermal equivalents: contribution to tissue organization by adaptation of myofibroblastic phenotype and function. Differentiation 2008;76(2):156-167

[96] Iwano M, Plieth D, Danoff TM, Xue C, Okada H & Neilson EG. Evidence that fibroblasts derive from epithelium during tissue fibrosis. The Journal of Clinical Investigation 2002;110(3):341-350

[97] Yu W, Ruest LB & Svoboda KK. Regulation of epithelial-mesenchymal transition in palatal fusion. Experimental Biology and Medicine (Maywood) 2009;234(5):483-491

[98] Potenta S, Zeisberg E & Kalluri R. The role of endothelial-to-mesenchymal transition in cancer progression. British Journal of Cancer 2008;99(9):1375-1379

[99] Kisseleva T & Brenner DA. Mechanisms of fibrogenesis. Experimental Biology and Medicine (Maywood) 2008;233(2):109-122

[100] Guarino M, Tosoni A & Nebuloni M. Direct contribution of epithelium to organ fibrosis: epithelial-mesenchymal transition. Human Pathology 2009;40(10):1365-1376

[101] Pisoschi C, Stănciulescu C, Munteanu C, Fusaru AM & Baniță M. Evidence for epithelial mesenchymal transition as a pathogenic mechanism of phenytoin induced gingival overgrowth. Farmacia 2012;60(2):168-176

[102] Zavadil J & Böttinger EP. TGF-beta and epithelial-to-mesenchymal transitions. Oncogene 2005;24(37):5764-5774

[103] Bolos V, Jorda M, Fabra A, Portillo F, Palacio J & Cano A. Genetic profiling of epitelial cells expressing E-cadherin repressors reveals a distinct role for Snail, Slug and E47 factors in epithelial-mesenchymal transition. Cancer Research 2006;66:9543-9556

[104] Kantarci A, Sume SS, Black SA, Lee A, Xydas C, Hasturk H & Trackman P. Epithelial and Connective Tissue cell CTGF/CCN2 Expression in Gingival Fibrosis: Role of Epithelial-Mesenchimal Transition) in CCN proteins in health and disease: An overview of the Fifth International Workshop of the CCN family of genes, Perbal A, Takigawa M & Perbal BV, Springer, 2010

[105] Holbourn KP, Acharya KR & Perbal B. The CCN family of proteins: structure-function relationships. Trends in Biochemical Sciences 2008;33(10):461-473

[106] Pisoschi CG, Stănciulescu CE, Munteanu C, Andrei AM, Popescu F & Baniță IM. Role of Transforming Growth Factor β – Connective Tissue Growth Factor Pathway in Di-hydropyridine Calcium Channel Blockers-Induced Gingival Overgrowth. Romanian Journal of Morphology and Embyology 2014;56(2):285-290

[107] Kisseleva T, Uchinami H, Feirt N, Quintana-Bustamante O, Segovia JC, Schwabe RF & Brenner DA. Bone marrow-derived fibrocytes participate in pathogenesis of liver fibrosis. Journal of Hepatology 2006;45(3):429-438

[108] Moore BB, Kolodsick JE, Thannickal VJ, Cooke K, Moore TA, Hogaboam C, Wilke CA & Toews GB. CCR2-mediated recruitment of fibrocytes to the alveolar space after fibrotic injury. The American Journal of Pathology 2005;166(3):675-684

[109] Quan TE, Cowper SE & Bucala R.The role of circulating fibrocytes in fibrosis. Current Rheumatology Reports 2006;8(2):145-150

[110] Hashimoto N, Jin H, Liu T, Chensue SW & Phan SH. Bone marrow-derived progeni-tor cells in pulmonary fibrosis. The Journal of Clinical Investigation 2004;113(2): 243-252

[111] Sakamoto R, Nitta T, Kamikawa Y, Kono S, Kamikawa Y, Sugihara K, Tsuyama S & Murata F. Histochemical, immunohistochemical, and ultrastructural studies of gingi-val fibromatosis: a case report. Medical Electron Microscopy 2002;35(4):248-254

[112] Häkkinen L & Csiszar A. Hereditary gingival fibromatosis: characteristics and novel putative pathogenic mechanisms. Journal of Dental Research 2007;86(1):25-34

[113] Almeida JP, Coletta RD, Silva SD, Agostini M, Vargas PA, Bozzo L &, Graner E. Pro-liferation of fibroblasts cultured from normal gingiva and hereditary gingival fibro-matosis is dependent on fatty acid synthase activity. Journal of Periodontology 2005;76(2):272-278

[114] Secombe J, Pierce SB & Eisenman RN. Myc: a weapon of mass destruction. Cell 2004;117(2):153-156

[115] Ridley AJ. Life at the Leading Edge. Cell 2011;145(7):1012-1022

[116] Quaggin SE & Kapus A. Scar wars: mapping the fate of epithelial-mesenchymal-my-ofibroblast transition. Kidney International 2011;80(1):41-50

[117] van Meeteren LA & ten Dijke P. Regulation of endothelial cell plasticity by TGF-β. Cell Tissue Research 2012;347(1):177-186

[118] Tomasek JJ, Gabbiani G, Hinz B, Chaponnier C & Brown RA. Myofibroblasts and mechano-regulation of connective tissue remodelling. Nature Reviews Molecular Cell Biology 2002;3(5):349-363

[119] Hinz B, Phan SH, Thannickal VJ, Galli A, Bochaton-Piallat ML & Gabbiani G. The myofibroblast. One function, multiple origins. The Americal Journal of Pathology 2007;170(6):1807-1816

[120] Tang WW, Van GY & Qi M. Myofibroblast and alpha 1 (III) collagen expression in experimental tubulointerstitial nephritis. Kidney International 1997;51(3):926-931

[121] Serini G & Gabbiani G. Mechanisms of myofibroblast activity and phenotypic modulation. Experimental Cell Research 1999;250(2):273-283

[122] Okada H, Danoff TM, Kalluri R & Neilson EG. Early role of Fsp1 in epithelial-mesenchymal transformation. The American Journal of Physiology 1997;273(4 Pt 2):F563-574

[123] Eyden B. The myofibroblast: an assessment of controversial issues and a definition useful in diagnosis and research. Ultrastructural Pathology 2001;25(1):39-50

[124] Desmoulière A, Chaponnier C & Gabbiani G. Tissue repair, contraction, and the myofibroblast. Review. Wound Repair Regeneration 2005;13(1):7-12

[125] Castella LF, Buscemi L, Godbout C, Meister JJ & Hinz B. A new lock-step mechanism of matrix remodelling based on subcellular contractile events. Journal of Cell Science 2010;123(Pt 10):1751-1760

[126] Lombardi T & Morgan PR. Immunohistochemical characterisation of odontogenic cysts with mesenchymal and myofilament markers. Journal of Oral Pathology & Medicine 1995;24(4):170-176

[127] Miguel MC, Andrade ES, Rocha DA, Freitas R de A & Souza LB. Immunohistochemical expression of vimentin and HHF-35 in giant cell fibroma, fibrous hyperplasia and fibroma of the oral mucosa. Journal of Applied Oral Sciences 2003;11(1):77-82

[128] Schor SL, Ellis I, Irwin CR, Banyard J, Seneviratne K, Dolman C, Gilbert AD & Chisholm DM. Subpopulations of fetal-like gingival fibroblasts: characterisation and potential significance for wound healing and the progression of periodontal disease. Oral Disease 1996;2(2):155-166

[129] Guo F, Carter DE & Leask A. Mechanical tension increases CCN2/CTGF expression and proliferation in gingival fibroblasts via a TGFβ-dependent mechanism. PLoS One 2011;6(5):e19756. doi: 10.1371/journal.pone.0019756

6

White Spots Lesions in Orthodontic Treatment and Fluoride — Clinical Evidence

Hakima Aghoutan, Sana Alami, Farid El Quars,
Samir Diouny and Farid Bourzgui

1. Introduction

Orthodontic treatment aims to improve functions and facial aesthetics by ensuring harmonious occlusal and jaw relationship; with beneficial effects on the oral health and quality of life of patients. However, it also associates risks and complications. Enamel surface demineralization or white spots lesions (WSL) remain by far one of the major adverse sequelae of fixed orthodontic appliance therapy, despite techniques and materials advances in preventive dentistry and orthodontics. They appear during and sometimes persist after orthodontic treatment; they can compromise the successful outcome of the treatment and result in the early termination of treatment. In severe cases of WSL, invasive interventions can be required and clinician responsibility may also be engaged.

WSL seem to be related to the interaction of several factors including inadequate elimination of dental plaque due to intrabuccal appliances that limit the self-cleansing mechanism of the oral musculature and saliva, patient's modifying factors and change in bacterial flora during fixed appliances wear. [1, 2]

Considering how quickly these lesions can develop, prevention, early diagnosis and treatment remain one of the greatest challenges facing orthodontists and requires a thorough knowledge of the caries disease and the risk factors specific to each patient. These risk factors should be accurately evaluated before and during any orthodontic treatment in order to minimize tooth decay and discoloration that could compromise the aesthetic of smile. Early detection of WSL during orthodontic treatment would allow clinicians to implement preventive measures to control the demineralization process before lesions progress.

The non-invasive prophylactic techniques are of critical importance during orthodontic treatment in order to decrease the incidence of demineralization. They involve either decreasing the amount of plaque by maintaining good dietary and oral hygiene, or tackling the susceptibility of enamel to demineralization [3]. Among suitable caries preventative agents, fluoride agents are usually used to reduce enamel decalcification and enhance its mineralization since fluoride contains bactericide and bacteriostatic properties.

The aim of this chapter is to outline the evidence regarding the effectiveness of fluoride administration in the prevention and management of WSL during orthodontic treatment.

2. White spot lesions in orthodontic treatment

WSLs have been defined as "subsurface enamel porosity from carious demineralization" that is located on smooth surfaces and presents as "a milky white opacity" [4] due to consequential changes in the optical properties of the enamel [1]. Various risk factors can contribute to the development of these incipient lesions. Poor oral hygiene, low salivary volume and a sugary diet promote the proliferation and activity of the microbial biofilm for a period of time. Orthodontic treatments are known as non-negligible factors and equal susceptibility has been reported whether teeth are banded or bonded.

The levels of oral bacteria have been reported to increase five folds upon the application of fixed bonds [5]. So orthodontic patients develop significantly more WSLs than non-orthodontic patients [1, 4]. The fitting of fixed orthodontic appliances (figure 1) (brackets, bands, arch wires, springs, elastomeric modules…) makes oral hygiene very difficult, restricts salivary self-cleaning and creates more stagnation areas for plaque; encouraging a lowering of plaque pH in the presence of carbohydrates and forming a physical barrier prevent remineralization by calcium and phosphate ions from the saliva. All these changes in the oral ecosystem favor colonization of aciduric bacteria, resulting in a rise in the levels of mutans streptococci and lactobacilli, mainly around the bonding adhesives [6, 7]. This can disrupt balance between the processes of demineralization and remineralization in favor of demineralization, and would lead to the permanent formation of white spot lesions. To these conditions, one must add the duration of orthodontic treatment: the longer the time of oral appliances' wearing is; the most prolonged the caries risk is. WSLs can develop into cavities and can no longer be reversed even in smooth surfaces that would normally have a low risk of caries [5, 8]. Tipping the balance back toward remineralization is the basis of WSL treatment although they can remain as cosmetic scars. However, even if high levels of mutans streptococci and lactobacilli in plaque indicate an increased risk of caries, the prediction of caries development based on bacterial counts is uncertain and it is of minor clinical significance [1, 9].

On the other hand, resting salivary flow rate rises during fixed appliance therapy; which increases salivary pH and buffer capacity and thus counteract the tendency for demineralization to occur around orthodontic appliances in some patients despite moderate plaque scores. This is especially true in individuals with good dietary regimen [5, 9]. Therefore, an assessment of patients' susceptibility In order to identify those most at risk of demineralization prior to

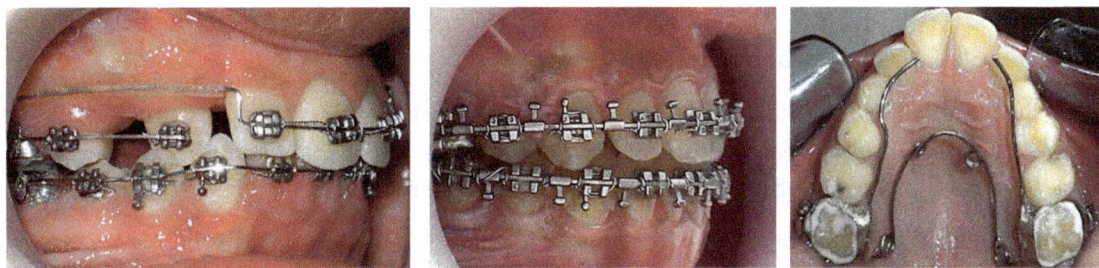

Figure 1. Fixed oral appliances increase stagnation areas of plaque and make oral hygiene difficult to carry out.

orthodontic treatment seems decisive. It was shown that subclinical demineralization before treatment may be a factor in the incidence of WSL during fixed appliance treatment [8].

In addition, orthodontic treatment is most often applied during adolescence, when the permanent teeth, recently erupted, are more vulnerable to caries because of their young enamel. Consequently, orthodontic treatment at this age will favor the formation of carious lesions in particular with the lack of cooperation encountered more frequently in this age group [10].

Commonly identified when the teeth are dry, WSL appears clinically as an opaque whitish or greyish halo under loose bands and around the bracket base periphery generally at the junction between the cement and the enamel, and at the gum level at the base of the half moon bracket (Figure 2). Studies show that these lesions can appear within a span of 4 weeks [11], which is even shorter than the time between two sessions of orthodontic appointments. Caries lesions may also develop after debonding in association with bonded retainer [1]. Furthermore, appliances' removing and tooth polishing cause a loss of the superficial enamel layer, rich in fluorine. This favors plaque retention due to porous enamel surface and thus decalcification. However, these alterations can gradually fade with natural abrasion and hygiene measures.

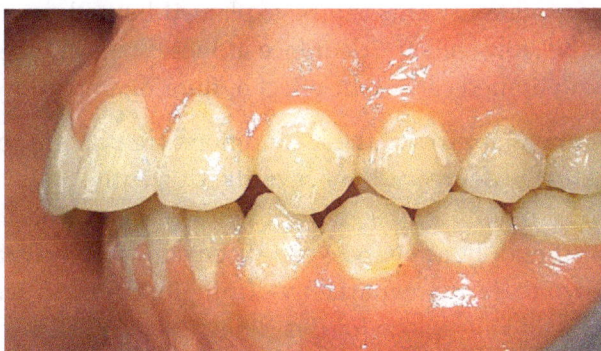

Figure 2. White spot lesions after orthodontic treatment localized at the gingival areas of teeth.

Since Zachrisson and Zachrisson (1971), WSL has been reported as a clinical observation [12]. Over the years, quantitative studies on decalcification incidence and prevalence have been reported. Depending on the examination technique used, the prevalence of WSL varies widely in the literature. It ranges from 23% and 89% when the teeth have been inspected using visual scales and photographic evaluation [8, 13-16].

Boersma et al. [16], using quantitative light fluoroscopy, investigated the prevalence of WSLs at the end of orthodontic treatment and reported that 97% of subjects had one or more lesions and on average, 30% of the buccal surfaces in a person were affected.

The large variation in reported prevalence may also be due to sample size disparity, the use or otherwise of a fluoride regimen during treatment and whether developmental or not other idiopathic enamel lesions, which artificially increases the prevalence quoted, are included or excluded [18].

Clinical studies [8, 13, 15, 19] have showed a sharp increase in the number of WSL during the first 6 months of treatment that continued to rise at a slower rate to 12 months; supporting the idea that the presence of fixed orthodontic appliances and greater treatment lengths serve as a risk factor for WSL formation. Hence, oral hygiene status of patients should be evaluated during the initial months of treatment and, if necessary, measures to prevent demineralization should be implemented.

With regard to the location of these lesions, studies have shown a significant increase in the prevalence on the cervical and middle thirds of the crowns. But they can broadly extend over the teeth surface and sometimes involve proximal extensions. The teeth most vulnerable to demineralization are the first permanent molars, the maxillary incisors, the mandibular lateral incisors and canines [1, 16, 18]. Premolars have also been reported to have greater frequency of WSL [8], and the lowest incidence was in the maxillary posterior segment. According to Samawi 2005 [In 18], upper anterior teeth showed larger mean demineralization surface area than anterior teeth in the lower arch; and the distogingival quadrant was particularly more affected than the mesiogingival quadrant in the upper lateral incisor teeth.

In a study conducted by Arneberg and coworkers [20], the bonded upper incisors have presented the lowest levels of total plaque fluoride and the lowest PH (as low as 4) during resting and fermenting conditions. This can be explained by both a prolonged retention of acids in plaque due to the slow salivary clearance at these sites, and also by loss of fluoride reservoirs associated with limited cariostatic effect of fluoride under low PH.

Regardless of WSL treatment approach, these conditions are difficult to treat and recover to some extent depending on the degree of their severity. Currently, there is a lack of conclusive long-term studies on WSL modifications after orthodontic treatment, but some clinical data can be stated. Once the orthodontic appliances have been removed and oral hygiene is restored, the area of WS was shown to decrease markedly during the first and second years following treatment [21, 22]. The most likely reason for this clinical healing can be explained by removal of the primary etiologic factor which is the cariogenic plaque adhered to fixed orthodontic elements, combined with enamel surface wear during tooth brushing and also by remineralization [1, 22]. However, some spots secondary to debonding can last from 6 to 12 years [22, 23] and ddo not not reach the pre-treatment level even 12 years after debonding [22]. Natural remineralization through saliva, involving mineral gain in the surface layer of WSL, has little improvement on the aesthetics and structural properties of the deeper lesions [24]. Evidence of success is characterized clinically by the recuperation of hardness and shine, whereas translucency is not always recovered. Indeed, WSL can take up stain and become discolored after many years. Therefore, it is necessary to apply remineralizing agents as early as possible for better aesthetic results.

3. Fluoride in management of orthodontic-related white spot lesions

Patients wearing orthodontic appliances are considered as patients at risk, for whom a preventive approach should be implemented before, during and after orthodontic treatment. Controlling risk factors, in addition to awareness of bucco-dental hygiene, and early diagnosis of WSL are key elements of success to reduce their prevalence and incidence during orthodontic treatment.

Both office-applied and self-care programs have been described for preventive and curative approaches of WSL. In self-administered programs, compliance has been identified as a significant problem.

Little information is available about measures that are really used in orthodontic practices to prevent and treat demineralization. But several procedures have been described in association with oral-hygiene instructions and patients' motivation. Reducing enamel susceptibility to demineralization by periodical professional fluoride application and varnishing reside at the bottom of the intervention hierarchy, and therefore represents the frontline of incipient caries treatment.

Actually, it has been known for many years that fluoride reduces the incidence of dental caries by maintaining the plaque fluoride supersaturated with respect to Fluor apatite, hence tipping the balance of the caries process in favor of remineralization. While full mineral recovery might be achieved through fluoride measures in the case of shallow enamel lesions in both children and adults, long-existing white spot lesions have demonstrated negligible remineralization after further contact with fluorides [25]. Upon failure of remineralization measures by fluoride agents in active lesions, other conservative procedures, such as resin sealing, have been advocated as alternative measures to prevent demineralization progression and cavitation.

There are two main methods of fluoride administration. However, there is little evidence about which fluoride supplement provides the greatest decrease in decalcification: In topical form, active ingredients are supplied in forms such as a toothpaste, mouth rinse, gel, varnish, mousse, pastille, or by adding it to chewing gum. Professionals usually apply gels and varnishes, particularly if they contain a high concentration of fluoride, whereas the other means of topical application can be self-administered. The second way is the use of materials containing the active ingredient fluoride as part of the appliance, either as a bonding or banding material, or an auxiliary such as a glass bead or elastic [3].

When topical fluoride is applied, a calcium fluoride-like material (CaF_2) builds up in plaque, on the tooth surface or in incipient lesions. The CaF_2 acts as a reservoir of fluoride ions for release when pH is lowered during a carious attack. When associated with phosphate ions,

CaF2 becomes more soluble and release fluoride at higher rate than the pure substance [1]. The preventive effect of fluoride can be illustrated using the Stephan curve (Figure 3). The limit of the fluoride effect is reached when pH drops below 4.5 so the solubility product of pure Fluor apatite is exceeded and no remineralization occurs. In old, acidic plaque a dose response to fluoride may not be apparent against lesion progression due to the low pH [26].

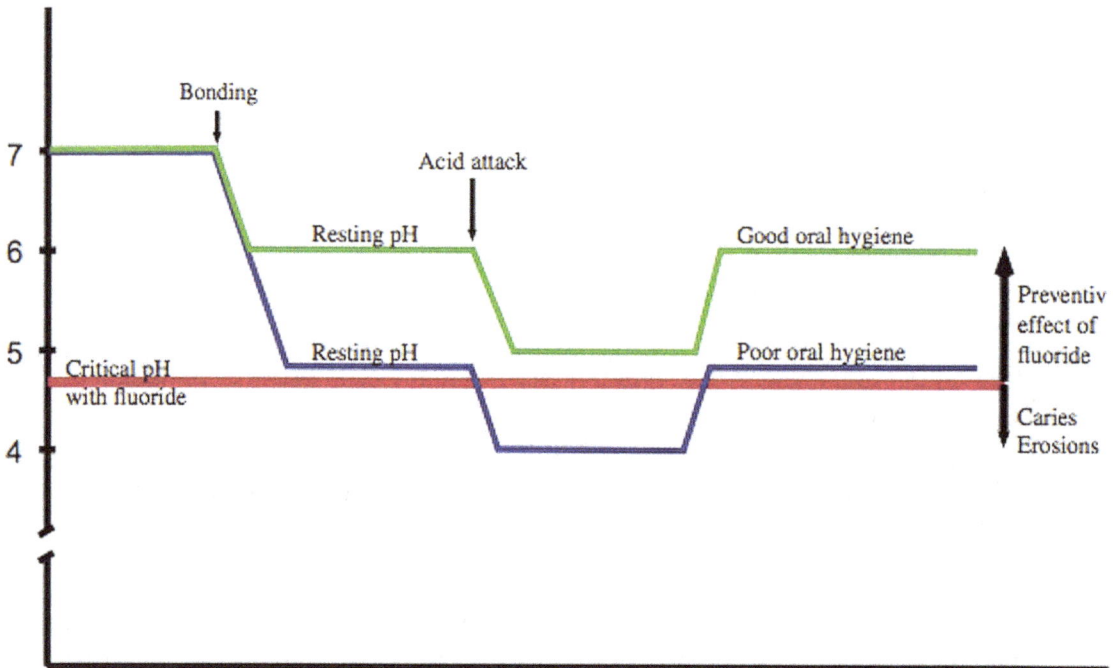

Figure 3. The Stephan curves in orthodontic patients with good or bad oral hygiene. After bonding, resting pH is lowered. An acid attack lowers the pH in the patient with bad oral hygiene below the critical pH of enamel. Assuming fluoride is frequently used, the critical pH of enamel is around 4.5 compared with 5.5 in the absence of fluoride. In the patient with good oral hygiene, fluoride is able to prevent lesions to develop. [1]

All these findings make optimal oral hygiene a crucial element that should be associated with fluoride prevention against WSL. Orthodontist must be cautious to create more favorable conditions to implement good oral hygiene by patients. Hence, the close fitting of bands on teeth is recommended and all excess bonging material around the attachment base should be eliminated. Also excessive surplus orthodontic etching of the complete labial enamel surface, instead of the bracket bases only, must be avoided to prevent iatrogenic white spot lesions [27], and steel ligatures or self-ligating brackets must be preferable to elastic ligatures [28]. (Figure 4)

According to Øgaard [1, 26], it is logical to differentiate between prevention of caries lesion development during orthodontic treatment and treatment of lesions present on labial surfaces at debonding. Clinical approaches differ in the two situations.

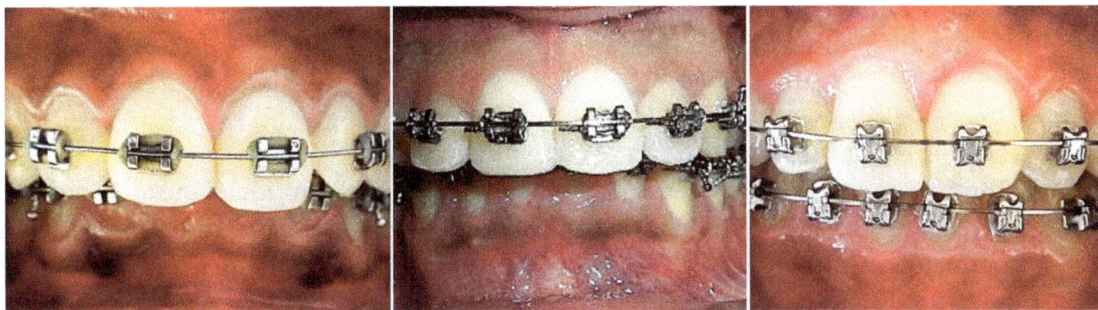

Figure 4. Different styles of ligatures: elastic ligatures (left) tend to discolor and increase the risk of plaque aggregation.

3.1. Fluoride prevention during orthodontic treatment

3.1.1. Oral-hygiene instructions

Clinical maintenance by elimination of plaque and food debris is essential throughout any orthodontic treatment as there is a much stronger relationship between oral hygiene and caries incidence in orthodontic patients than in non-treated individuals [26]. Therefore satisfactory level of oral hygiene should be successfully maintained despite the hindrance of the appliance.

Among the self-applied fluoride products available, toothpaste used in tooth brushing is thought to be the most important. Fluoridated toothpaste exerts a cariostatic effect. It increases fluoride levels in the biofilm, where it acts as an inhibitor of bacterial enzymes, and can reduce the frequency of caries by 15–30% [29]. Authors [30] have emphasized the need for at least two daily brushings in order to favor a continuous exchange of fluoride ions between the salivary and the enamel surface. The availability of fluoride from toothpaste is influenced by several factors, such as the concentration of fluoride, the amount of toothpaste used, and the post-brushing behavior (Davies and Davies, 2008; Zero et al., 2010 (In [31]). The fluoride concentration in toothpaste has traditionally been limited to 1450 ppm F; but in multicenter randomized controlled trial [31], authors have reported that daily use of high-fluoride (5000ppm) toothpaste may be recommended to prevent WSL during fixed oral appliances. This corroborates with other studies [32] that stipulate that the relative caries preventive effects of fluoride toothpastes of different concentrations increase with higher fluoride concentration. Fluoride concentrations below 0.1% should not to be recommended for orthodontic patients [1].

The daily use of a fluoride mouth rinse throughout brace treatment to prevent WSL is also highly recommended [33-34]. It was demonstrated that the daily use of a 0.05% sodium fluoride rinse during orthodontic treatment resulted in a statistically significant reduction of enamel white spot lesions. The more closely patients adhered to this rinsing regimen the more likely they exhibited a decrease in the occurrence of white spot lesions. The dose response effect between the frequency of rinsing and the incidence of white spots was evident regardless of oral hygiene status [34]. Besides self-controlled oral hygiene, professional prophylactic cleaning using fluoridated pastes is designed to reduce bacterial load and enhance the efficacy of brushing mainly in difficult areas around appliances [35].

3.1.2. In office-applied topical fluorotherapy

Use of additional topical fluorides designed to deliver additional fluoride to the tooth surface at-risk area near orthodontic brackets is likely to reduce the risk of DWL development. In a review conducted in 2103 [36], the authors found some moderate evidence that fluoride varnish applied every six weeks at the time of orthodontic review during treatment is effective. It has also been reported that the application of a fluoride varnish resulted in a 44.3% reduction in enamel demineralization in orthodontic patients [37], and there were significantly fewer new demineralized white lesions in the patients that had the application of the fluoride varnish at each visit compared with the placebo varnish [38].

Additionally, with in office-applied fluoride varnishes, the amounts of fluoride exposure can be controlled better and does not depend on patients' compliance. However, there is a limitation on the frequency of fluoride exposures received since the application occurs in the clinician's office only. In addition, the repeated varnish applications may lead to the temporary discoloration of the teeth and gingival tissue, and increase costs to the patient and/or chair time to the clinician [4]. In order to enhance the cariostatic potential of current fluoride agents and procedures for orthodontic purposes, substance like titanium fluoride or stannous fluoride has been described to reduce lesion depths and total mineral loss when compared to conventional fluoride preparations. The acid resistant coating deposited from these solutions can protect the enamel surface against severe acid challenges from plaque with low pH [1, 39, 40] (Figure 5).

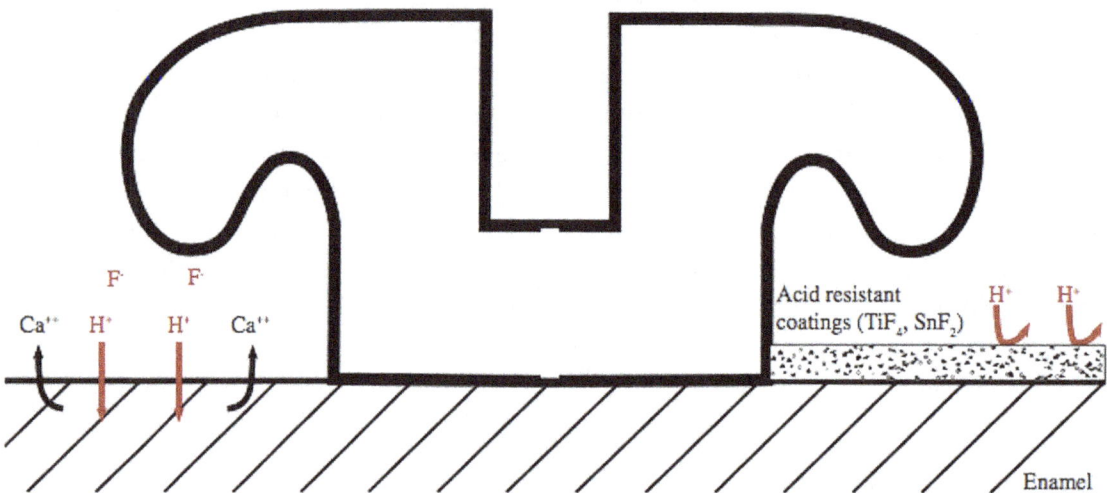

Figure 5. Acid resistant coating deposited from titanium fluoride or stannous fluoride, protect the enamel surface against severe acid challenges (H^+ions under the right bracket wing). Conventional fluoride preparations have a reduced cariostatic effect in plaque with low pH (under the left bracket wing). Ca^{2+}loss illustrates the caries process [1].

The use of antimicrobials like Chlorhexidene, as a complement to fluoride therapy, has also demonstrated demineralization-inhibiting tendencies in patients with fixed orthodontic appliances to reduce WSL at the time of debonding when compared with a control group [1, 4, 23, 26]. Chlorhexidene varnishes for long-term use may reduce the cariogenic challenge sufficiently to improve the fluoride effect on WSL instead daily Chlorhexidene rinsing, which is a well-known cause of teeth and tongue discoloration [23]. In this context, the use of products combining fluorides and antimicrobial agents should be seriously considered, especially among patients with a lack of motivation to maintain optimal oral hygiene, provided that such products do not significantly decrease mechanical properties of the adhesive system used [4].

On the other hand, if fluoride use may be beneficial for WSL prevention during orthodontic treatment, it can have conversely unwanted effects on properties of orthodontic alloys. In the presence of fluoride, β titanium, currently used for his elasticity and corrosion resistance, can undergo a degradation process and be affected in terms of biological and mechanical features. Thus, coating with TiAlN (deposing thin films of titanium aluminium nitride) has been recommended [41] in order to reduce the corrosive effects of fluorides on β titanium orthodontic archwires. Likewise, fluoride attacks the protective oxide surface film on Nickel-Titanium wires causing corrosion and nickel release, which increases with increasing fluoride concentration [42]. Some authors have recommended diamond-like carbon (DLC) coatings onto nickel-titanium wires to reduce fluoride-induced corrosion and improve orthodontic friction [43].

3.1.3. Fluoride-releasing materials used in orthodontic practice

While compliance with preventive protocols at home is the most frequently difficult to obtain [44], it would be an advantage if bonding materials could inhibit demineralization near the brackets. Presently, it seems impossible to make recommendations on the use of fluoride-containing orthodontic materials during fixed orthodontic treatment. However, it is advantageous to report some studies outcomes.

Using fluoride containing sealants and adhesives to bond brackets has been attempted. Glass ionomer cements (GIC) were initially introduced as orthodontic bonding adhesives for their ability to chemically bond to tooth structure and their sustained fluoride release following bonding. Resin particles were added to their formulation to create Resin-modified glass ionomer cements (RMGIC). These bonding systems have been developed to combine the desirable properties of composite resin bond strength and glass ionomer fluoride release. Studies have shown that RMGIC is more effective than an acrylic-bonding agent in preventing white spot formation, but weak evidence was reported [22, 45]. It has been suggested that these adhesives should be more widely used in bonding orthodontic brackets [46] particularly on the maxillary incisors that represent a significant aesthetic challenge to both the patient and the orthodontist.

Additionally, filled and fluoride releasing sealant may offer more enamel protection next to orthodontic brackets exposed to cariogenic conditions, mainly in patients with poor oral hygiene [47, 48]. Their application has been shown to not affect the shear bond strength (SBS) of orthodontic adhesives, and they are able to produce a sustained fluoride release [4, 42]. It was also found out that using the combination of an antimicrobial self-etching primer and a fluoride-releasing adhesive had acceptable bond strength for clinical use [49]. However, the clinical effectiveness of the fluoride release may be questionable, as the amount of fluoride required from a bonding material to be caries preventive is still unknown [50].

Resin composite bonding system with the ability of fluoride release was also developed for bracket bonding. An in-vitro study using nano-indentation test to evaluate the nano-mechanical properties of the enamel around and beneath orthodontic brackets, has showed that use of these product may reduce demineralization during orthodontic treatment [51].

3.2. Fluoride use after orthodontic treatment

The best treatment of WSL begins with a preventive approach, as they are difficult to recover especially in severe cases. In addition, White spot lesions treatment after appliance removal to produce a sound and aesthetically pleasing enamel surface is still a question to be fully answered. As patients respond differently to the presence of WSL, the course of treatment will likely be unique to each patient [4].

Debonding the orthodontic appliances eliminates an important cariogenic environment. However, the removal of stagnant plaque alone is not enough to achieve complete repair of WSL, and some spots secondary to debonding can last from 5 to 12 years [22, 52]. Evaluation of lesions that have developed during appliance therapy in the different sites of the dentition represents a clinical challenge for orthodontists [1]. Initial surface-softened lesions appear to remineralize quickly in saliva even without fluoride [53]. Resolution is thought to occur via the redisposition of various minerals soluble in saliva, particularly calcium, phosphate, and fluoride, but also and primarily via surface wear exposing the underlying enamel crystals, which are tightly packed and thus provide proper light reflection [54]. When arrested, they may exhibit a white color or may become yellowish or dark brown due to exogenous uptake of stains.

In general, treatment of WSL should begin with the most conservative approaches. If such approaches do not resolve the problem to the clinician's satisfaction, more aggressive treatment modalities can be pursued if the patient is interested (micro-abrasion, composite restorations, tooth whitening, porcelain veneers….)

Although the treatment of post-orthodontic WSL differs from their prevention, topical fluoride is thought to be the first step in WSL management. Based on the literature, and compared with the evidence on the WSL forestalling during orthodontic treatment, there is a lack of reliable evidence to support the effectiveness of remineralizing agents for the treatment of post-orthodontic white spot lesions [52, 55-56]. Nevertheless, for mild WSL, application of lower concentrations of fluorides can be used in an attempt to arrest their progression with successful and more aesthetic treatment results since hypermineralization maintains the whiteness of the lesions. Indeed, direct application of a high concentration of fluoride is not recommended as it causes rapid remineralization of the enamel surface, which restricts the passage of ions into the deeper, more affected layers, and limits their complete recovery [4, 57].

Finally, it has been suggested that acid etching of WSLs may increase the surface porosity and hence remineralization [1]. However, a study by Al-Khateeb et al (2000) [58] has shown lack of complete remineralization, and the etched lesions retained a porous structure of their surface layer even after a long period of remineralization in vitro.

4. Experience of Casablanca Dental School in fluoride use during orthodontic treatment

A clinical study was conducted for 10 months and 3 days in the Department of Dento Facial Orthopedics at the Faculty of Dentistry in Casablanca to determine the incidence of WSL in orthodontic population and to evaluate the fluoride varnish effect on the prevention and remineralization of carious lesions generated by orthodontic treatment.

5. Method framework

All patients starting treatment at the Dentofacial Orthopedics Unit from December 2010 to April 2011 were selected. The survey included healthy patients aged from 12 to 27 years old, and for whom treatment duration was estimated at more than 6 months. Patients with anterior restorations (composite, glass ionomer, endodontic treatment) or prosthetic devices, those displaying tooth tissue abnormalities (fluorosis, amelogenesis imperfecta, WSL....) or following preventive fluoride regimens (except toothpaste) and those with orthodontic treatment history were excluded. A total of 68 consecutive orthodontic patients fulfilled the eligibility criteria and were approached to participate.

This was a prospective study that has been made in the form of Crossover, which exposes teeth to the same factors: Oral hygiene, saliva composition, and enamel's structure. All patients were fitted with multi-bracket appliance and the same bonding system. The right side, from the central incisor to the first molar, has received a fluoride varnish (Fluor Protector 0, 1% F, Ivoclar Vivadent, Schaan, Liechtenstein) while the left side was taken as control. Before applying the varnish, an evaluation of oral hygiene status was recorded via plaque quantification for each tooth in both lower and upper arch. WSL were evaluated by naked eye after teeth brushing and drying with air spray, and scored depending on their severity and location according to the modified White spot lesion index (WSL-Index) by Gorelick et al. (1982) [59]. The visual evaluation of the individual teeth was based on a labial surface examination assessing the presence or absence of WSL. The severity of WSL was scored as follows: (Figure 6, 7)

(0)=No white spot lesion formation

(1)=Slight white spot or line formation

(2)=Excessive white spot formation

(3)=White spot formation with cavitations

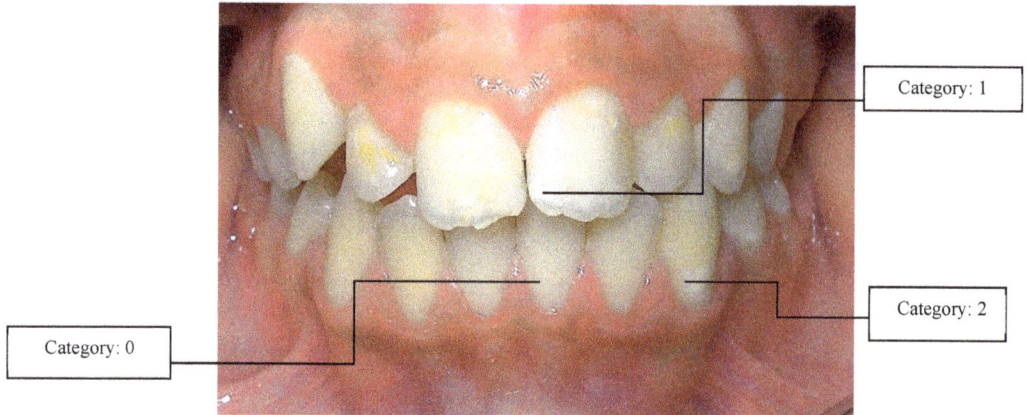

Figure 6. Evaluation of WSL 0, 1 and 2

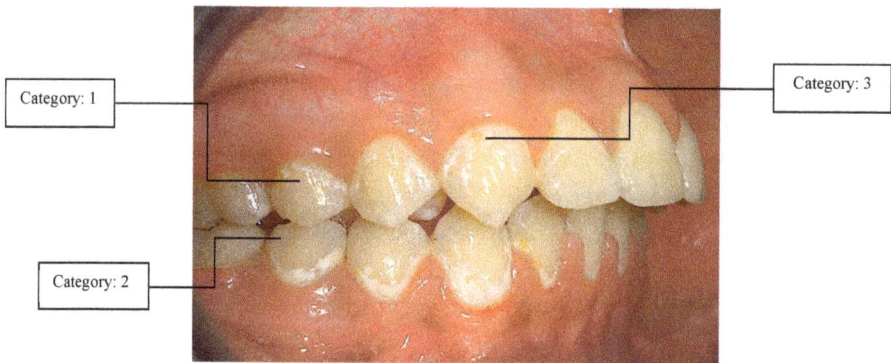

Figure 7. Evaluation of WSL 1, 2 and 3

Patients were notified about the importance of complying with the recommendations advocated by the manufacturer: Avoid eating and brushing teeth for 45 min after the application of fluoride varnish. The varnish was applied every 6 weeks for a six-month period. After every 6 weeks, the plaque index and the WSL formation have been evaluated for all the teeth in two arches.

In total, we conducted 5 applications of fluoride varnish during the 6 months of the study. The statistical analysis of the data was performed using the software Epi6.0 fr.

6. Results

From 68 selected, only 30 patients have been recruited for the study. 38 were excluded from the study because they did not respect their periodic appointments, they did not show up

The sample study was distributed as follows: (figure 8-10)

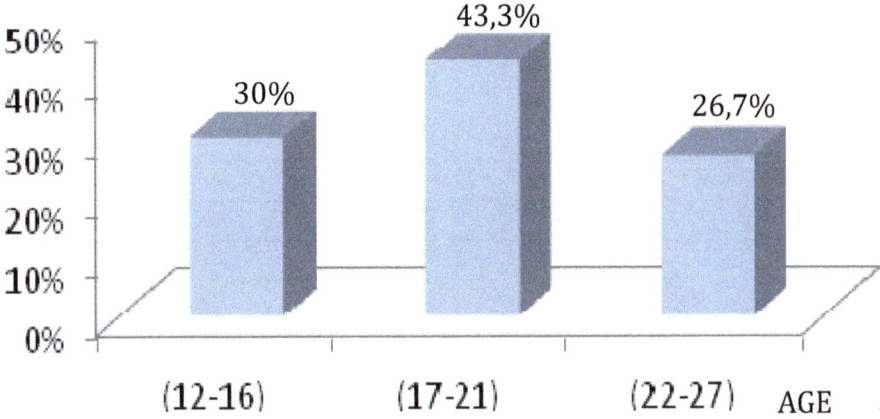

Figure 8. Sample distribution by age

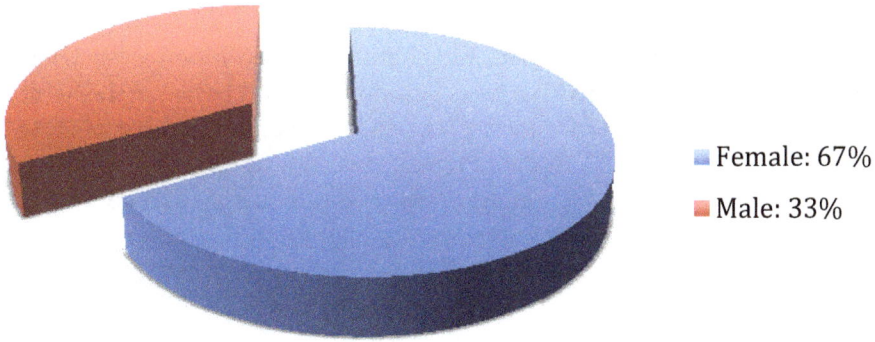

Figure 9. Sample distribution by sex

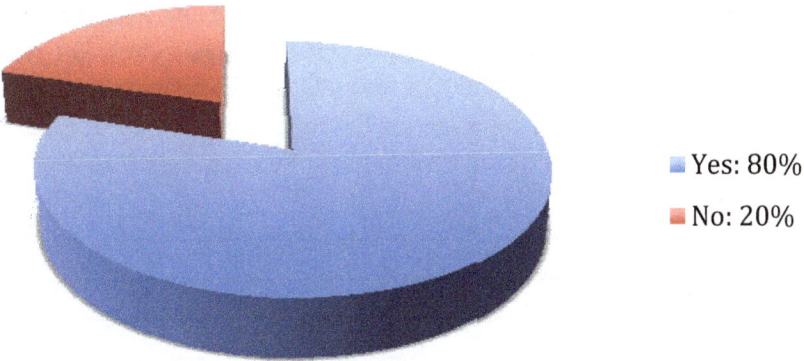

Figure 10. Sample distribution according to the sugary diet

Oral hygiene was evaluated by the frequency and method of brushing as well as the amount of plaque (table 1). The vertical brushing method was the most used by study's patients, and 73, 3% used no way adjuvant for their daily tooth brushing. According to the saliva parameters, 76, 7% of patients had a normal salivation and 63, 3% had fluid saliva.

Plaque	Appointment n°1		Appointment n°2		Appointment n°3		Appointment n°4		Appointment n°5	
	Number	%	Number	%	Number	%	Number	%	Number	%
0≤P<1	15	50, 0	15	50, 0	18	60, 0	20	66, 7	21	70, 0
1≤P<2	12	40, 0	11	36, 7	12	40, 0	9	30, 0	9	30, 0
P≥2	3	10, 0	4	13, 3	0	0, 0	1	3, 3	0	0, 0
Total	30	100	30	100	30	100	30	100	30	100

Table 1. Distribution of the study's sample according to the plaque amount

In the test group of teeth, the incidence of WSL was 60% versus 66.7% in the control group. In addition, 55.5% of female patients and 44.5% of male patients have developed WSL against 56, 5% and 43, 5% respectively in the control group.

On the other hand, 73.7% patients with snacking habit have developed at least one WSL versus 72, 7% in those without this practice. No association was found between the habit of snacking and the appearance of WSL. The frequency of people who had at least one WSL increases according to the number of snack, but the difference was not significant (table 2). Likewise and paradoxically, there was more WSL among those without sugary diet compared with those who consumed more sweet foods, but the difference was not significant. The saliva parameters have also been considered. The X^2 test (P=0. 71) has shown no association between the quality and the quantity of saliva and the appearance of WSL (table 3-4).

Both in the group of teeth test than in the control group, there was at baseline more of WSL among patients with mediocre and average oral hygiene compared with those who had good hygiene. By the end of the study, the opposite was observed. But in both cases, the difference was not significant.

As for varnish effect, there were fewer WSL in the teeth having benefited from fluoride varnish compared with the contralateral, but the difference was not significant. The relative risk was 0.73 with a confidence interval of [0.49-1.09]. It was < 1, which seems to be in favor of fluoride varnish. This reflects that fluoride is a protective factor, but we cannot draw any conclusions conclude on the basis of the results of the confidence interval of the relative risk (table 5).

Snacks number	0		1		2		3	
	Number	%	Number	%	Number	%	Number	%
WSL presence	8	72.7%	8	72.7%	6	85.7%	0	0, 0%
WSL absence	3	27.3%	3	27.3%	1	14.3%	1	100, 0%
X^2 = 3, 30		p = 0, 34				No significant difference		

Table 2. Association between snacks number and WSL formation

	Hyper salivation		Normal salivation	
	Number	%	Number	%
WSL presence	5	71.4%	17	73.9%
WSL absence	2	28.6%	6	26.1%
X² = 0, 02	p = 0, 62		No significant difference	

Table 3. Association between saliva quantity and WSL formation

	Viscous Saliva		Fluid Saliva	
	Number	%	Number	%
WSL presence	8	72.7%	14	73.7%
WSL absence	3	27.3%	5	26.3%
X² = 0, 14	p = 0, 71		No significant difference	

Table 4. Association between saliva quality and WSL formation

	WSL presence	WSL absence	Total
Test group	33	172	205
Control group	46	163	209
X² = 0, 92	p = 0, 12	No significant difference	

Table 5. Evaluation of the occurrence of WSL

7. Discussion

During this investigation, we have tried to avoid bias in order to obtain valid results and overcome some difficulties regarding:

- The lack of cooperation and refusal of participation of some patients.
- The lack of reliability concerning oral hygiene and dietary habits.
- The non-respect of appointments
- Gingival inflammation of the maxillary premolars after the brackets location and poor hygiene. So the cervical zone was often weakly induced by fluoride varnish.

7.1. Discussion of the findings

As discussed above, identification of risk factors of carious lesions is a necessary step before any orthodontic treatment is undertaken. In this respect, dietary habits are of great importance.

Beyond the amount of sugar ingested, the frequency of the daily ingestion maintains oral PH in critical levels, and thus, leads to the development of the caries process.

A study conducted on 155 patients in the Department of Dentofacial Orthopedics at Casablanca Dental Schoolto evaluate the prevalence of dental caries and associated risk factors in orthodontics (Bourzgui et al, 2010) [60], showed that 31, 6% of patients had an excessive sugary diet and 45, 8% had a snack habit. In the present investigation, this estimation was 80% and 63, 3%, respectively. However, the association between WSL formation and the dietary habits (number of meals, snacking and consumption of sugary diets)was not significant.

The fitting of orthodontic appliances causes adverse changes in the composition of the bacterial plaque increasing radically periodontal and caries risk. Adolescents following orthodontic treatment are considered to be high-risk patients and they need more motivation, hygiene control and use of topical fluoride [61]. Good individual control of dental plaque associated with a daily use of topical fluoride per toothpaste remains the most effective way. Patients with good oral hygiene during fixed orthodontic treatment have less prevalence of enamel decalcification. Simple daily oral hygiene procedures have shown a reduction in these decalcifications. Four factors influence the effectiveness of oral brushing: The frequency of brushing, brushing length, the concentration of fluoride and rinse after brushing. Oral brushing should be done at least twice a day and for a longer duration. The high fluoride concentration toothpaste is recommended. The use of fluoride supplementation (fluoride mouthrinse, varnishes, gel…) is of great interest to prevent WSL and reduce their severity [62]. Our study has shown a slight improvement in the frequency of brushing (43.3% brushed three times per day at the beginning of the investigation versus 53.3% at the end) with a non-significant difference between the WSL occurrence and the brushing frequency.

Additionally, all teeth have presented at least one demineralization except the first right upper Premolar. However, some patients presented a total lack of demineralization. The previous study conducted in the same Dental Clinic [60] showed that 7.7% of patients developed whit spots during their orthodontic treatment, with a similar distribution between front and posterior areas of the arches. Our study has shown that the most affected tooth in the control group was the first molar, followed by upper lateral incisor, upper cuspid, and then premolar group. While in the experimental group, the lateral incisor was the most affected, followed by canines, and the premolar group (Figures 11-12). The lateral incisors in some cases had a palatine position at the base, and they thereby were subject concurrently to the fastest accumulation of plaque due to the cleaning difficulty.

In the literature, all the studies conducted so far have used different fluoride concentration with different application frequencies (Table 6). The findings consolidated the use of topical fluorides in addition to fluoride toothpaste as the best evidence-based way to forestall these incipient lesions. Regular high fluoride varnish application around the brackets is the most effective topical method. It is a quick and easy professional application with conservation and a slow-release fluoride for an extended time period. Also, it is usefully independent of patients' compliance [63]. In our study, the incidence of whit lesions in the control group was slightly higher than the test group. However, the chi-2 test was not significant, so according to our study, there was no association between the application of fluoride varnish and the appearance of whitish lesions; this could be explained by the fact that our sample was small and the duration of our study was short. In this study, fluoride varnish reduced the severity of lesions, but it did not prevent their appearance.

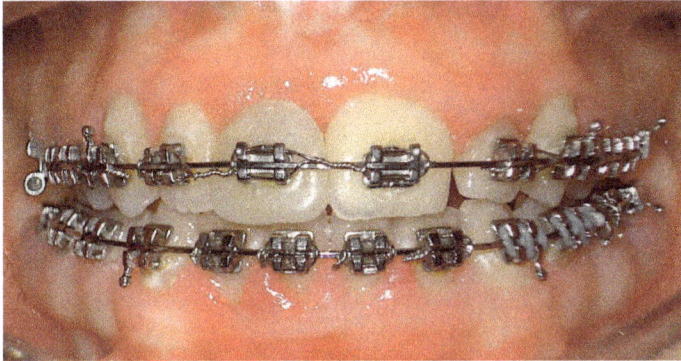

Figure 11. WSL on cervical area on lower and upper incisors and cupids during orthodontic treatment.

Authors (year)	Sample	Fluoride varnish	Frequency	Results	Incidence Test/ control
Gontijo (2007)	16 teeth	Duraphat 22600 ppm	One application	Significant Difference in the composition of enamel	-
Farhadian (2008)	15 patients	Bifluoride: 12, 6% of calcium flourideand 6% of sodiumfluoride	One application	Significant difference	57/93
Stecksén-Blicks (2004)	273 patients	Fluor Protector 1000ppm	Every 6 weeks	Significant difference	7/26
Vivaldi-Rodrigues (2006)	10 patients	-	Every 3 months	Significant difference	0, 34/0, 51*

*Index of decalcification

Table 6. Examples of in vivo studies about WSL prevention

The secondary prevention, that is the control and treatment of existing WSL after debonding, has gained interest, too. Treatment of post-orthodontic WSL, with a remineralizing cream with casein phosphopeptide-stabilized amorphous calcium phosphate (CPP-ACP) as adjunct to fluoride toothpaste seemed to be beneficial with some mineral and aesthetic improvements compared with fluoride applications [63].

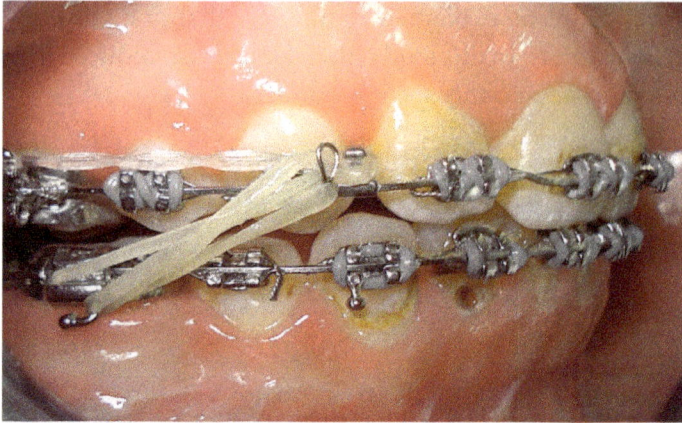

Figure 12. Development of a cavity in cervical zone of the 43 during orthodontic treatment

While the findings of the different studies areequivocal, further research with standardized protocols, is needed before practice guidelines on the fluoride/non-fluoride therapies can be recommended.

8. Conclusion

Even with the advances in material and techniques, demineralization around brackets during orthodontic treatment remains problematic. The literature points to the need for more evidence to clarify the most recent opinions, on which orthodontists can base their clinical practice. Developing a practice and standardized guideline for the prevention and the treatment of enamel demineralizations at the start of, during, and after orthodontic treatment is highly recommended to improve outcomes quality and manage unplanned debondings.

There are a number of products containing fluoride available to clinicians and their patients. Unfortunately, the evidence for the effectiveness of these products is weak. However, to date, using fluoride varnish in high concentration and with regular applications is the most effective way to avoid WSL appearance. This should be implemented in close association with the control of caries risk factors. Indeed, It is still crucial to emphasize that prevention of these lesions is the furthermost desirable outcome aesthetically and also the least costly for patients.

As for treatment of WSL already installed, the concerns are more complicated. It is expected that the majority of slight or mild the WSL will improve during the retention period if good oral hygiene is maintained. For more advanced cases, total recovery remains unsystematic. The lesions may induce aesthetic consequences and require more invasive approaches. However, current evidence supports the use of topical application of fluoride in low concentration or better the use of CPP-ACP to obtain a reduction in the severity of these lesions.

Author details

Hakima Aghoutan[1], Sana Alami[1], Farid El Quars[1], Samir Diouny[2] and Farid Bourzgui[1*]

*Address all correspondence to: faridbourzgui@gmail.com

1 Department of Dento-facial Orthopedic, Faculty of Dental Medicine, Hassan II University of Casablanca, Morocco

2 Chouaib Doukkali University, Faculty of Letters & Human Sciences, El Jadida, Morocco

References

[1] Øgaard B. White spot lesions during orthodontic treatment: mechanisms and fluoride preventive aspects. Seminars in Orthod. 2008; 14(3): 183-93.

[2] Hadler-Olsen S, Sandvik K, El-Agroudi MA et al. The incidence of caries and white spot lesions in orthodontically treated adolescents with a comprehensive caries prophylactic regimena prospective study. Eur J Orth 2012; 314 : 633-39

[3] Benson PE. Prevention of Demineralization during orthodontic treatment with fluoride-containing materials or casein phosphopeptide-amorphous calcium phosphate. In Huang GJ, Richmond S, Vig KWL.(eds) Evidence-Based Orthodontics. Blackwell Publishing, Ltd 2011 p149-65

[4] Bishara SE, Ostby AW. White Spot Lesions: Formation, Prevention, and Treatment. Semin Orthod 2008;14:174-82

[5] Chang HS, Walsh LJ, Freer TJ. Enamel demineralization during orthodontic treatment. Aetiology and prevention. Aust Dent J. 1997; 42(5): 322-7.

[6] Jung WS, Kim H, Park SY, et al. Quantitative analysis of changes in salivary mutans streptococci after orthodontic treatment. Am J Orthod Dentofacial Orthop. 2014; 145(5): 603-9.

[7] Lim BS, Lee SJ, Lee JW et al. Quantitative analysis of adhesion of cariogenic streptococci to orthodontic raw materials. Am J Orthod Dentofacial Orthop. 2008; 133(6): 882-8.

[8] Chapman JA, Roberts WE, Eckert GJ et al. Risk factors for incidence and severity of white spot lesions during treatment with fixed orthodontic appliances. Am J Orthod Dentofacial Orthop. 2010; 138(2): 188-94.

[9] Van Palenstein Helderman WH, Matee MI, van der Hoeven JS, et al. Cariogenicity depends more on diet than the prevailing mutans streptococcal species. Dent Res. 1996; 75(1): 535-45.

[10] Kukleva M P, Shetkova D G, Beev V H: Compara-tive age study of the risk of demin-eralization during orthodontic treatment with brackets. Folia Med 2002; 44: 56-9.

[11] Øgaard B, Rølla G, Arends J: Orthodontic appliances and enamel demineralization. Part 1. Lesion development. Am J Orthod Dentofacial Orthop 1988; 94: 68-73.

[12] Zachrisson BU, Zachrisson S. Caries incidence and orthodontic treatment with fixed appliances. Scand J Dent Res 1971; 79: 183-92.

[13] Julien KC, Buschang PH, Campbell PM. Prevalence of white spot lesion formation during orthodontic treatment. Angle Orthod. 2013; 83: 641-47.

[14] Lovrov S, Hertrich K, Hirschfelder U. Enamel demineralization during fixed ortho-dontic treatment—incidence and correlation to various oral-hygiene parameters. J Orofac Orthop. 2007; 68: 353-63.

[15] Tufekci E, Dixon JS, Gunsolley JC, Lindauer SJ. Prevalence of white spot lesions dur-ing orthodontic treatment with fixed appliances. Angle Orthod. 2011; 2: 206-10.

[16] Khalaf K. Factors affecting the formation, severity and location of white spot lesions during orthodontic treatment with fixed appliances. J Oral Maxillofac Res 2014; 5(1): e4. 10.5037/jomr.2014.5104

[17] Boersma JG, van der Veen MH, Lagerweij MD, et al. Caries prevalence measured with QLF after treatment; with fixed orthodontic appliances: influenc-ing factors. Ca-ries Res. 2005; 39: 41-7.

[18] Willmot D. White Spot Lesions After Orthodontic Treatment. Semin Orthod 2008;14: 209-19.

[19] Lucchese A, Gherlone E. Prevalence of white-spot lesions before and during ortho-dontic treatment with fixed appliances. Eur J Orthod. 2013; 35(5): 664-8.

[20] Arneberg P, Giertsen E, Emberland H, et al: Intra-oral variations in total plaque fluo-ride related to plaque pH. A study in orthodontic patients. Caries Res 1997; 31: 451-56.

[21] Mattousch TJ, van der Veen MH, Zentner A. Caries lesions after orthodontic treat-ment followed by quantitative light-induced fluorescence: a 2-year follow-up. Eur J Orthod 2007; 29: 294-8.

[22] Shungin D, Olsson AI, Persson M. Orthodontic treatment-related white spot lesions: a 14-year prospective quantitative follow-up, including bonding material assessment. Am J Orthod Dentofacial Orthop 2010; 138: 136-7.

[23] Øgaard B, Larsson E, Henriksson T, et al: Effects of combined application of antimi-crobial and a fluoride varnishes in orthodontic patients. Am J Orthod Dento-facial Orthop 2001; 120: 28-35.

[24] Cochrane NJ, Cai F, Huq NL, et al. New approaches to enhanced remineralization of tooth enamel. J Dent Res 2010; 89: 1187-97.

[25] Belli R, Rahiotis C, Schubert EW, Baratieri LN et al. Wear and morphology of infiltrated white spot lesions. J dentistry 2011; 39: 376–85

[26] Øgaard B: Oral microbiological changes, long-term enamel alterations due to decalcification, and caries prophylactic aspects, in Brantley WA, Eliades T, eds: Orthodontic Materials. Scientific and Clinical Aspects. Stuttgart, Thieme, 2001, p123-142

[27] Knösel M, Bojes M, Jung K, et al. Increased susceptibility for white spot lesions by surplus orthodontic etching exceeding bracket base area. Am J Orthod Dentofacial Orthop 2012;141:574-82.

[28] Garcez AS, Suzuki SS, Ribeiro MS, et al. Biofilm retention by 3 methods of ligation on orthodontic brackets: a microbiologic and optical coherence tomography analysis. Am J Orthod Dentofacial Orthop. 2011; 140 (4): e193-8.

[29] Derks A, Katsaros C, Frencken JE, et al. Caries-inhibiting effect of preventive measures during orthodontic treatment with fixed appliances: a systematic review. Caries Res 2004; 38: 413-20.

[30] Farhadian N, Miresmaeili A, Eslami B, at al. Effect of fluoride varnish on enamel demineralization around brackets: an in-vivo study. Am. J. Orthod. Dentofacial Orthop. 2008; 133: S95-98.

[31] Sonesson M, Twetman S, Bondmark L. Effectiveness of high-fluoride toothpaste on enamel demineralization during orthodontic treatment: a multicenter randomized controlled trail. Eur J Orth. 2013; Dec 28 doi: 10.1093/ejo/cjt096.

[32] Walsh T1, Worthington HV, Glenny AM, et al. Fluoride toothpastes of different concentrations for preventing dental caries in children and adolescents. Cochrane Database Syst Rev. 2010; 20(1):CD007868. doi: 10.1002/14651858.CD007868.pub2.

[33] Geiger AM, Gorelick L, Gwinnett AJ, Benson BJ. Reducing white spot lesions in orthodontic populations with fluoride rinsing. Am J Orthod Dentofacial Orthop 1992; 101: 403-7

[34] Kerbusch AE, Kuijpers-Jagtman AM, Mulder J, Sanden WJ. Methods used for prevention of white spot lesion development during orthodontic treatment with fixed appliances. Acta Odontologica Scandinavica 2012; 70(6): 564–8.

[35] Arnold WH, Dorow A, Langenhorst S et al. Effect of fluoride toothpastes on enamel demineralization. BMC Oral Health 2006; 6(8): 1-6.

[36] Benson PE, Parkin N, Dyer F, et al. Fluorides for the prevention of early tooth decay (demineralised white lesions) during fixed brace treatment. Cochrane Database of Systematic Reviews 2013 (12). Art. No.: CD003809. DOI: 10.1002/14651858.CD003809.pub3.

[37] Vivaldi-Rodrigues G, Demito CF, Bowman SJ, et al: The effectiveness of a fluoride varnish in preventing the development of white spot lesions. World J Orthod. 2006; 7:138-44.

[38] Stecksen-Blicks C, Renfors G, Oscarson ND. et al. Caries-preventive effectiveness of a fluoride varnish: a randomized controlled trial in adolescents with fixed orthodontic appliances. Caries Research 2007; 41: 455-59

[39] Buyukyilmaz T, Tangugsorn V, Øgaard B, et al: The effect of titanium tetrafluoride (TiF4) application around orthodontic brackets. Am J Orthod Dentofacial Orthop, 1994; 105: 293-96.

[40] Hove L, Holme B, Øgaard B, et al: The protective effect of TiF4, SnF2 and NaF on erosion of enamel by hydro-chloric acid in vitro measured by white light interferometry. Caries Res 2006; 40: 440-43.

[41] Krishnan V, Krishnan A, Remya R, et al. Development and evaluation of two PVD-coated ß-titanium orthodontic archwires for fluoride-induced corrosion protection. Acta Biomater. 2011; 7(4): 1913-27

[42] Brantley WA. Wires used in orthodontic practice. In Miles PG, Rinchuse DJ, Rinchuse DJ (Eds) Evidence-based clinical orthodontics. 2012 Quintessence Publishing Co Inc

[43] Huang SY, Huang JJ, Kang T, et al. Coating NiTi archwires with diamond-like carbon films: reducing fluoride-induced corrosion and improving frictional properties. J Mater Sci Mater Med. 2013; 24 (10): 2287-92.

[44] Geiger AM, Gorelick L, Gwinnett AJ, et al. Reducing white spot lesions in orthodontic populations with fluoride rinsing. Am J Orthod Dentofacial Orthop 1992; 101: 403-7.

[45] Rogers S, Chadwick B, Treasure E. Fluoride-containing orthodontic adhesives and decalcification in patients with fixed appliances: a systematic review. Am J Orthod Dentofacial Orthop. 2010; 138(4): 390.e1-8

[46] Eliades T: Orthodontic materials research and applica-tions: Part 1. Current status and projected future devel-opments in bonding and adhesives. Am J Orthod Dentofacial Orthop 2006; 130:445-51

[47] Hu W, Featherstone JD. Prevention of enamel demineralization: an in-vitro study using light-cured filled sealant. Am J Orthod Dentofacial Orthop. 2005; 128(5): 592-600

[48] Behnan SM, Arruda AO, Gonzàlez-Cabezas C, et al. In-vitro evaluation of various treatments to prevent demineralization next to orthodontic brackets. Am J Orthod Dentofacial Orthop 2010; 138: 712.e1-712.e7.

[49] Korbmacher HM, Huck L, Kahl-Nieke B: Fluoride-releasing adhesive and antimicrobial self-etching primer effects on shear bond strength of orthodontic brackets. Angle Orthod. 2006; 76:845-50.

[50] Pseiner BC, Freudenthaler J, Jonke E, et al. Shear bond strength of fluoride-releasing orthodontic bonding and composite materials. Eur J Orthod. 2010; 32(3): 268-73.

[51] Raji SH, Banimostafaee H, Hajizadeh F. Effects of fluoride release from orthodontic bonding materials on nanomechanical properties of the enamel around orthodontic brackets. Dent Res J. 2014; 11(1): 67–73.

[52] Chen H, Liu X, Dai J, et al. Effect of remineralizing agents on white spot lesions after orthodontic treatment: A systematic review. Am J Orthod Dentofacial Orthop. 2013; 143(3): 376-82.e3.

[53] Øgaard B, ten Bosch JJ: Regression of white spot enamel lesions. A new optical method for quantitative longitudinal evaluation in vivo. Am J Orthod Dentofacial Orthop 1994; 106 : 238-42.

[54] Artun J, Thylstrup A. A 3-year clinical and SEM study of surface changes of carious lesions after inactivation. Am J Orthod Dento-facial Orthop 1989; 95: 327-33.

[55] Kalha AS. Lack of reliable evidence of the effectiveness of remineralising agents for the treatment of post orthodontic white spot lesions. Evid Based Dent. 2013; 14(3): 76-7.

[56] Ballard RW, Hagan JL, Phaup AN, et al. Evaluation of 3 commercially available materials for resolution of white spot lesions Am J Orthod Dentofacial Orthop. 2013; 143: S78-84.

[57] Artun J, Thylstrup A. Clinical and scanning electron microscopic study of surface changes of incipient caries lesions after debonding. Scand J Dent Res 1986; 94: 193-201.

[58] Al-Khateeb S, Exterkate RAM, Angmar-Månsson B, et al: Effect of acid-etching on remineralization of enamel white spot lesions. Acta Odontol Scand 2000; 58:31-6.

[59] Gorelick L, Geiger AM, Gwinnett AJ. Incidence of white spot formation after bonding and banding. Am J Orthod. 1982; 81: 93-8.

[60] Bourzgui F, Sebbar M, Hamza M. Risk of caries in orthodontics: descriptive study on 155 patients. Rev Stomatol Chir Maxillofac. 2010; 111: 276-79.

[61] Chaussain C, Opsahl Vital S, Viallon V, et al. Interest in a new test for caries risk in adolescents undergoing orthodontic treatment. Clin Oral Investig. 2010; 14: 177–85

[62] Al Mulla AH, Kharsa SA, Birkhed D. Modified fluoride toothpaste technique reduces caries in orthodontic patients: A longitudinal, randomized clinical trial. Am J Orthod Dentofac Orthop. 2010; 138: 285-91

[63] Bergstrand F, Twetman S. A review on prevention and treatment of post-orthodontic white spot lesions–evidence based methods and emerging technologie. Open Dent J. 2011; 5: 158-62.

7

Salivary Diagnostics, Current Reality and Future Prospects

Andréa Cristina Barbosa da Silva, Diego Romário da Silva,
Sabrina Avelar de Macedo Ferreira, Andeliana David de Sousa Rodrigues,
Allan de Jesus Reis Albuquerque and Sandra Aparecida Marinho

1. Introduction

1.1. Saliva: Composition and functions

Saliva is a aqueous, transparent and odorless liquid produced and secreted by the major and minor salivary glands, which combined with the gingival crevicular fluid, cellular debris, upper airway secretions and microorganisms of the oral cavity, makes up the total human saliva [1, 2].

The saliva is responsible for maintaining the homeostasis of the oral cavity and its pH normally lies around 6-7, which makes it slightly acidic. Initially, it shows up isotonic, becoming hypotonic as it passes through the network of ducts [3].

The daily average flow of total saliva in healthy people varies between 500 and 1500 mL, and the mean volume of saliva in the oral cavity is approximately 1 mL; however, there is always a great variability in individual rates of salivary flow [3]. This flow provides important information about the health quality not only oral but also systemic [4, 5].

The main constituent of saliva is water, which accounts for 99% of its composition. Solid components, which are characterized by organic and inorganic molecules, are dissolved in the aqueous medium. The salivary composition has significant changes from one individual to another and in the same individual under different circumstances; however, the rate of salivary flow is considered the main factor affecting its composition [6].

Saliva is composed of a number of inorganic ions, including sodium, potassium, chloride, calcium, magnesium, bicarbonate, phosphate, sulfate, thiocyanate and fluoride, which are responsible for osmotic balance, buffering capacity and dental remineralization [7]. Humphrey and Williamson (2001), [3] consider that bicarbonate, phosphate and urea act as pH modulators being responsible for salivary buffering capacity.

The salivary organic components are represented by immunoglobulins, proteins, enzymes, mucins, and nitrogen products such as urea and ammonia. The salivary proteins (amylase, lipase, proteases, nucleases, mucins and gustin) act assisting in the digestive process, with antibacterial properties for hydrolysis of cellular membranes (lactoferrin, lysozyme and lactoperoxidase) besides inhibiting the adherence of microorganisms (immunoglobulins) [7].

The saliva keeps the oral health and creates a proper ecological balance. Among its functions (Figure 1) are the protection and lubrication of oral tissues, acting as a barrier against irritants, with buffering and cleaning action, maintaining the integrity of the teeth and antibacterial activity, besides acting improving the taste and starting the digestive process [8]. The saliva's lubricity capacity is provided mainly by mucins, they are secreted by the minor salivary glands, having low solubility, high viscosity, high elasticity and strong adhesiveness [6, 9, 10].

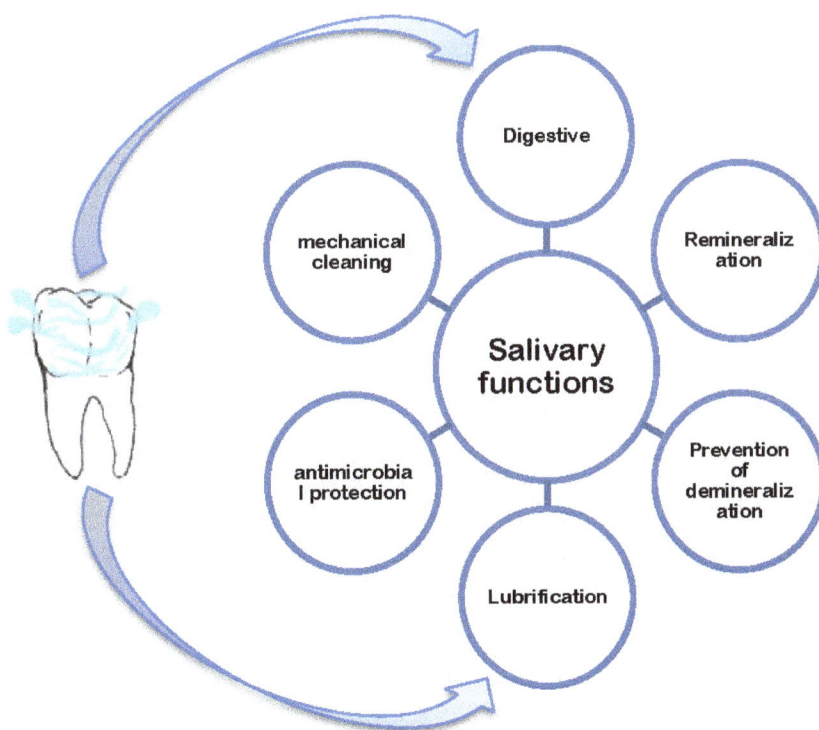

Figure 1. Saliva functions

Saliva was used for a long time as a method to monitor the caries risk, being used as biological environment extremely useful as buffering capacity and microbiological evaluation. Today, it is an object of detailed study for the diagnosis of systemic diseases that affect the function of the salivary glands and saliva composition, for example, Sjögren's syndrome, alcoholic cirrhosis, cystic fibrosis, sarcoidosis, diabetes mellitus and adrenal cortex diseases [11, 12]).

According to [13], saliva is a valuable source of clinically relevant information, since its many components, besides protecting the oral tissues integrity, act as biomarkers of diseases and systemic conditions of the individual. The qualitative changes in the composition of these biomarkers have been used to identify patients with increased susceptibility to some diseases, identification of sites with active disease, prediction of sites with greater disease activity in the future and / or serving as a tool for monitoring effectiveness of therapies.

2. The role of salivary biomarkers for diagnosis

There have been significant advances in techniques for detection of biomarkers in the oral cavity in recent years, especially by ELISA for proteins and PCR for RNA and DNA. With these advances in biotechnology, it has become possible to use saliva as a diagnostic mean for different conditions such as caries and periodontal disease, infectious and autoimmune diseases, genetic and psychological disorders, malignancies, legal issues, among others (Figure 2).

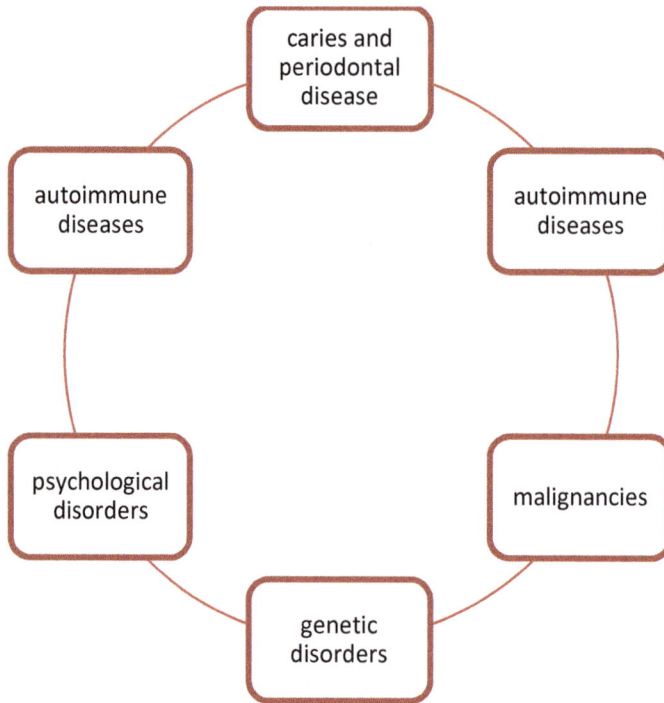

Figure 2. Major diseases with possibility of salivary diagnostics.

2.1. Caries and periodontal disease

Caries [14] and periodontal disease [15]) are the most occurring diseases in the oral cavity. Both considered infectious diseases and primarily responsible for tooth loss in adults. In recent years, remarkable achievements have been made in the field of oral microbiology, especially with regard to diagnosis. Techniques have been sought to predict the availability of patients to certain diseases; and this is not different with caries. The counts of bacteria present in saliva associated with other factors, such as diet and systemic conditions, may provide an estimate of the risk of caries in the individual. The increased number of lactobacilli and *Streptococcus mutans* in saliva have been associated with increased prevalence of caries and root caries [16]. Similarly, the methods of diagnosis in current clinical practice are able not only to detect the presence of inflammation, but also to identify patients at higher risk for progression of periodontal disease [17].

The human salivary buffer systems consist of an important natural defense against tooth decay [18]. The saliva's buffer capacity varies with glandular activity. The bicarbonate raises the pH of saliva and its buffering capacity, especially during stimulation [19]). Thus, the levels of bicarbonate and other important ions showing abnormalities can also suggest a predisposition to dental caries.

There has been an association between periodontal disease and increased levels of aspartate aminotransferase (AST) and alkaline phosphatase (ALP). The salivary AST can be used as a marker for monitoring periodontal disease. In addition, lower uric acid levels and albumin in saliva were associated with periodontitis and diabetes [20]. The development of new devices for periodontal monitoring probably would require less training and fewer resources than current diagnostic tests and may lead to better use by properly trained professionals for simpler and less intensive treatment, and may result in the provision of health care at low cost [21]. For determination of periodontal disease, it would be necessary a large body of research previously focused on fluid gingival biomarkers that provide the local disease status, but represents a technically difficult approach to implement in the clinical area [13, 17].

Currently, it is possible to use saliva tests for evaluating the microbiota associated with periodontal diseases, regardless of the degree of periodontal impairment of the patient. PCR tests can detect DNA of periodontal bacteria in oral fluids, such as *ggregatibacter actinomyce-temcomitans*, *Porphyromonas gingivalis*, *Campylobacter rectus*, *Eikenella corrodens* and *Fusobacterium nucleatum*. The analysis of the salivary microbial content reflects periodontal conditions and various socio-economic, cultural and behavioral aspects of patients [22].

2.2. Infectious diseases

In addition to exercising extremely important functions for the organism's homeostasis, saliva is currently an important tool for the diagnosis of infectious diseases. Besides the usual microorganisms in oral cavity, saliva may contain viruses and/or bacteria responsible for systemic diseases that can be identified by PCR. Another way to diagnose infectious disease by the salivary examination is through monitoring the presence of antibodies to the organisms [23].

Today, it is possible to identify, for example, the herpes virus associated with Kaposi's sarcoma and the presence of bacteria such as *Helicobacter pylori*, which is associated with gastritis, peptic ulcers and possible stomach cancer [11, 12]. Studies conducted in order to detect immunoglobulin M (IgM) against rubella showed 96% specificity when compared to standard considered as ideal test blood serum, which means that the use of saliva for epidemiological surveillance and control of this virus can be valid [24, 25]. It is also possible to detect the presence of Epstein-Barr virus (EBV) associated with infectious mononucleosis, highly communicable disease by contacting saliva and hairy leukoplakia [26].

The disease that generates more discussion regarding the use of saliva for diagnostic procedures is undoubtedly the Acquired Immunodeficiency Syndrome (AIDS). Until recently, oral HIV transmission through saliva of infected individuals during dental treatment or as a result of biting or contact stemmed by cough or kiss droplets has been considered less likely than vaginal or rectal transmission [27]. However, concerns about the way of transmission have increased. Studies have shown that these tests based on specific salivary antibodies are equivalent in reliability as compared to those in the serum, therefore being useful in the clinical use and epidemiological studies [28]. In recent years, researchers have shown that salivary tests for detection of antibodies to HIV [29] represents a non-invasive alternative for quantification of antibodies in blood to monitor the effectiveness of antiretroviral therapy and progression of Acquired Immunodeficiency Syndrome [30].

2.3. Autoimmune diseases

For this class of diseases, the most studied in parameters of salivary diagnostics is the Sjogren's syndrome. It is an autoimmune disease characterized by decreased secretion of the salivary and lacrimal glands, associated with endocrine disorders. The sialochemistry (analysis of saliva's chemical components) offers great value for the diagnosis of this syndrome. Increased immunoglobulin levels, inflammatory mediators, albumin, sodium and chloride and, decreased phosphate level are indicative of Sjögren's syndrome. Analysis of proteins in saliva showed increased level of lactoferrin, beta 2 microglobulin, lysozyme C, and cystatin C. However, levels of salivary amylase and carbonic anhydrase showed reduced [31, 32]. Thus, these references of protein chemical analysis associated with detailed history may show effectiveness for an accurate diagnosis.

Salivary changes that may reveal the presence of multiple sclerosis, an inflammatory disease characterized by loss of myelin and scarring caused due to failure in producing cells by the immune system have also sought. However, no significant changes were found except for a reduction in the production of IgA, which is inconclusive to suggest the diagnosis [33].

Sarcoidosis is an autoimmune and inflammatory disease, which affects the lymph nodes, lungs, liver, eyes, skin, or other tissues. Salivary diagnostics has demonstrated a decreased amount of saliva secretion associated with reduced activity of the enzyme alpha-amylase and kallikrein in most patients carrying the disease. However, there was no correlation between the decrease in enzyme activity and the volume of secretion, which complicates the understanding of salivary changes and possible diagnosis [34].

2.4. Psychological and genetic disorders

The total salivary flow and its characteristics had already been correlated with xerostomia, symptoms of anxiety, depression, Burning Mouth Syndrome and aphthous stomatitis [35, 36, 37]. The salivary cortisol levels may represent an important biological marker of stress. The salivary cortisol concentration increases after 20 the beginning of a stressful situation, besides increased pH and protein levels. However, there are no indications of changes in concentrations of fluoride under conditions of acute mental stress [38, 39].

The sialochemistry evaluation reveals significant elevation in the levels of phosphate, chloride and potassium in subjects with BSA symptoms, and also differences in expression pattern of salivary proteins of low molecular weight compared to healthy individuals. Levels of phosphate, potassium and chloride are increased in individuals with intense activity of the sympathetic nervous system, something common in situations of emotional stress [40].

The salivary alpha-amylase has its release regulated by the sympathetic autonomic nervous system, and has importance in the psychobiology of stress. The levels of salivary alpha-amylase in humans increase under various conditions of physical and psychological stress before any other clinical signs can be perceived [37, 41, 42]. Therefore, the salivary alpha-amylase may act as effective biomarker which can be used alternatively non-invasive way to evaluate psychological and metabolic stress, or including diseases whose etiology just seems to be related to stress.

Results are controversial and not always enlightening. For aphthous stomatitis significant changes in the levels of TCD4+ and TCD8+ lymphocytes have been associated and abnormal cytokine cascade arising from the oral mucosa. It is known that for aphthous stomatitis there are 41 genes expressed differently and increased activity of lymphocytes T-helper 1 (Th1), responsible for the production of interferon-gamma, interleukin 2 (IL-2) and alpha tumor necrosis factor (TNF-α). The levels of IL-2 are higher in patients with aphthous stomatitis compared with control subjects and may serve as markers in immunodiagnoses [43, 44, 45, 46, 47].

The secretory immunoglobulin A (IgA-s) can be used as the oral mucosa immune status parameter. It acts as a barrier to infectious agents, environmental allergens and carcinogens, as well as it participates in innate protection mechanisms. IgA deficiency is the most common humoral immune defect in humans and causes, in a large proportion, gastrointestinal and respiratory infections [48, 49, 50, 51].

The identification of exogenous genetic material in saliva may have forensic significance, or in cases of sexual assaults. The genetic material shared after a kiss is present and can be detected up to an hour after the kiss [52].

Cystic fribose, an autosomal recessive genetic disease caused by a disturbance in salivary glands secretions. Cystic fibrosis affects the chromosome 7, which is responsible for the production of a protein which will regulate the passage of sodium and chloride throuh cell membranes. The effects of this regulation can be analyzed through saliva. The Sodium and Potassium elements showed higher levels, while the trace elements vanadium, chromium, selenium and arsenic have lower levels in individuals with cystic fibrosis [53].

2.5. Malignancy

There is a growing interest worldwide for the saliva analysis through genomics, transcriptomics and proteomics, since this is a non-invasive source of rich genetic information. In the case of saliva, two main aspects of cancer diagnosis must be distinguished - one being the diagnosis of oral cancer (which has direct contact with saliva) and other the cancer diagnoses in other locations. Mouth cancer in advanced stages can usually be detected by inspection of the oral cavity. On the other hand, initial oral carcinomas are not visible and cannot be diagnosed and treated on time. The salivary proteome can also be used for tumor detection [54].

The study of Streckfus et al. (2000) [55], demonstrated the role of saliva in the diagnosis of breast cancer, in which salivary tests for markers of disease were studied combined with mammography. From the analysis in saliva, the soluble fragment of the oncogene c-erbB-2, a prognostic marker for breast cancer, as well as the antigen for cancer were significantly higher in the saliva and serum of women diagnosed with cancer than that observed in a control group of healthy women and patients with benign tumors group, indicating that the saliva test for this oncogene is sensitive and reliable, and it is potentially useful in the early detection and monitoring of screening for breast cancer [56].

Additionally, the use of saliva test may be important in monitoring the levels of c-erbB-2 in patients undergoing chemotherapy and/or surgery, so that serves as an assessment of therapy effectiveness in question, and may be useful in preservation [57].

Franzmann et al. (2005) [58], evaluated the soluble CD44 in saliva as a potential molecular marker for head and neck cancer and concluded that the test can be effective to detect this cancer at all stages.

In the past, biomarkers were used primarily as prognostic indicators for patients with tumors of the head and neck. More recently, the role of biomarkers has been greatly expanded to cover all aspects of patient care, from early cancer detection to the more accurate tumor staging and even the selection of those patients most likely to benefit from specific therapies to post-treatment tumor surveillance. One of the most promising avenues regarding the early diagnosis of cancer has been the ability to use saliva as a substrate for the evaluation of biomarkers [59].

Recently, Jiang et al. (2005)[60], reported increased content of mitochondrial DNA in saliva of patients with head and neck cancer. Multivariate analysis revealed a significant and independent association of SCC diagnosis of head and neck, age and smoking with increased content of mitochondrial or nuclear DNA. Salivary proteins such as CEA, defensin-1, TNF-alpha, IL-1, 6 and 8 and CD44 showed increase in their detection in patients with oral cancer.

Most of these studies relied on immunological assays of individual gene products 2,137. It is expected that proteomic biomarkers, when combined, increase the sensitivity and specificity of detection of human cancer [61, 62].

Increased levels of salivary defensin-1, CA15-3 cancer antigen, tumor marker proteins, such as c-erbB-2 or CA-125 and antibodies against tumor suppressor protein p53 are promising markers of oral malignant neoplasms and other cancers. In the future, a global proteomic profile of saliva with methods newly developed for proteome analysis is likely to result in other peptide sequences candidates for detection with high sensitivity [62, 54].

When compared to blood, saliva can express more sensitive and specific markers for certain local oral diseases. For example, saliva contains expressed proteins locally different from serum that can be best indicators of the oral disease. There are compelling reasons to use saliva as a diagnostic fluid to monitor the onset and progression of oral cancer. Saliva is the fluid that drains the lesions and there is increased RNA and proteins of oral cancer on it [63].

2.6. Forensic evidence

The forensic dentistry method is efficient for human identification, but is endowed with certain limitations: it suffers distortion from the moment of the bite until the act of expertise, especially when the mark is left on the skin. The salivary DNA emerges as a complement or even to replace the first, since it is a test of excellence [64]. However, the use of saliva in the identification was only feasible after the development of molecular biology techniques applied to forensic dentistry. In forensic uses, the PCR technique is the most used as it drastically increases the chances of DNA analysis, allowing determining the individual's molecular profile. It was from then that saliva became a great focus on looking for traces, as they provide enough genetic material and excellent qualities for the exam in most cases [65].

The DNA can be degraded depending on the conditions of their preservation. Moisture, excessive heat, pH, enzymes and other are variables for its ideal preservation under the various surfaces that can be found [66].This being the object of several recent studies. In the study by [67], the authors concluded that saliva is able to provide genetic material, even when stored under conditions below those considered optimal.

The human salivary proteome (HSP), using 2D gel electrophoresis coupled to mass spectrometry, is able to identify approximately 100 different salivary proteins [68]. A significant number of spots on a typical 2-DE gel can capture fragments of abundant salivary proteins such as amylases, cystatins and immunoglobulins [69]. For the identification of less abundant salivary proteins, analysis by advanced techniques of mass spectrometry ensures a significant increase in resolution when compared to two-dimensional gel electrophoresis [70]. Generally, a pre fractionation of intact salivary proteins employing high resolution separation techniques is required to achieve a wide coverage of the human salivary proteome [71].

Human saliva stains can be found at crime scenes, alone or mixed with other biological fluids. The most common sites of occurrence are: the surface of objects such as envelopes [72], tissues cigarette butts, cups, sites near bites and often victims of rape [73].

3. Clinical application of salivary diagnosis in the era of "omics"

For the salivary diagnosis become routine in clinical practice, it is necessary to know specific salivary biomarkers of disease states or health, besides technology necessary for their detection [74]. The genomics, epigenomics, transcriptomics, proteomics and metabolomics (Figure 3) approaches are currently being used to characterize these diagnostic biomarkers in saliva [75].

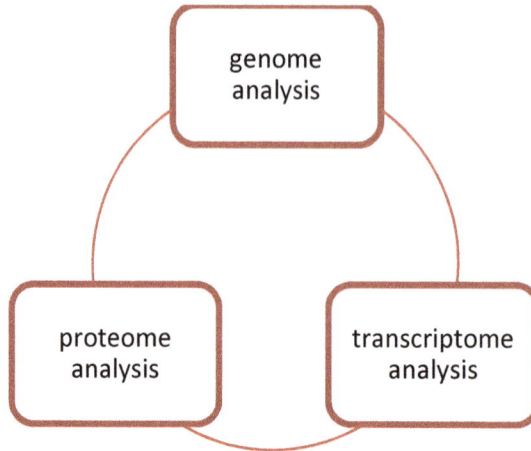

Figure 3. Study of omics to identify salivary biomarkers.

Biomarkers of DNA, mRNA, or protein biomarkers can provide useful diagnostic information that can identify the effect of disease or medication on salivary constituents. However, there is still not a complete characterization of the salivary proteome for disease biomarkers. Five hundred salivary proteins have been described, but this number is very small when compared to the more than 4,000 proteins listed for plasma [76].

The analysis of salivary genome and epigenoma allows identification of the presence of invading pathogens, as well as profiles transcription of anomalous genes that reflect genetic pathological processes such as cancer. The salivary genome consists of DNAs representing the individual's genome and the oral microbiota. The quality and yield of DNA that can be obtained from saliva is relatively good compared to blood and urine, which can be used for genotyping, amplification or sequencing [54], and can be stored for a long time without significant degradation [77].Thus, the salivary DNA is an analyte suitable for diagnosis but limited to reflect the presence or absence of specific genes or alterations in the sequences (mutations) and also cannot provide information about upregulation and downregulation of gene expression.

Regarding the salivary transcriptome, mRNAs and miRNAs are secreted by cells into the extracellular medium and can be found in biofluids remote cellular sources [78, 79, 80]. In the disease state, the transcription of specific miRNAs and mRNAs has changed. Despite suffering some criticism initially, the use of salivary RNAs as diagnostic biomarkers, is now widely accepted [81]. However, the precise sources of salivary RNAs and other molecules remain unclear.

The standard procedures for the isolation and analysis of salivary mRNA require low temperatures, besides being expensive and time consuming, precluding its clinical application. Currently, simple methods of stabilization of mRNA in saliva samples have been developed, allowing for storage at room temperature without the use of stabilizers, and are so-called 'direct-saliva-transcriptomic-analysis' [82]. However, this approach also involves centrifugation. An alternative method has been described [83], but it was based on the use of an expensive stabilizing agent (expensive). Thus, neither method is completely suitable for all applications. The mRNAs of saliva and plasma can be remarkably stable. The microarray technology is considered the gold standard for the identification of salivary transcripts. In this technique, the salivary transcriptome is determined using microarrays and is validated by means of qPCR. However, low concentrations of certain biomarkers, as well as small sample volumes require innovations in technology [84].

For proteins detection, the use surface - enhanced laser desorption/ionization time - of - flight (SELDI - TOF) mass spectrometry (MS), has been reported for several diseases. Recently, analysis of saliva for protein biomarker discovery has mainly been performed using two - dimensional difference gel electrophoresis (2D - DIGE) coupled with MS (which can identify around 300 proteins in a sample, and liquid chromatograpy - MS (LC - MS) based techniques (which can identify more than 1,050 proteins in a sample; reviewed in [85]. Thus, liquid chromatographic separation appears to resolve protein species more precisely than gel electrophoresis methods. A multiplex protein array was also employed, providing high - throughput analysis [86]; however, this method requires some prior knowledge of likely analytes. Despite these advances, the discovery and validation of protein salivary biomarkers still has some challenges. Proteins have short half-lives, making them unstable. Both the nature of peptides, as the oral environment makes them vulnerable to degradation. Thus, the diagnosis based on salivary protein requires immediate processing of samples, or the use of freezers and expensive protease inhibitors. In the clinical environment, these requirements are not easily circumvented.

The metabolome is the set of small metabolites and changes continuously, reflecting the gene and protein expression. Metabolomics investigations can generate quantitative data to elucidate metabolic dynamics related to disease and exposure to drugs [87]. However, a metabolomics limitation comparative to genomics, transcriptomics and proteomics is the inability to identify differentially the metabolites expressed [88, 89, 90].

4. Future prospects

In recent years, many important biological questions have been answered by the study of the "omics" (genomics, transcriptomics, proteomics, metabolomics, etc.), allowing the discovery of various salivary biomarkers. However, few of these markers have exceeded the identification phase. The transfer of scientific knowledge of salivary biomarkers for clinical applications is a challenging process that rarely has resulted in clinical implementation. Its successful application in clinical practice will depend on collaborative studies including physicians, epidemiologists, molecular biologists and bioinformaticians with a relevant clinical question and with well-defined parameters of recruitment and characterization of patients and samples. Thus, the use of saliva as a diagnostic fluid will be increasingly accepted, allowing for enhanced systemic and oral health.

Author details

Andréa Cristina Barbosa da Silva[1*], Diego Romário da Silva[1],
Sabrina Avelar de Macedo Ferreira[1], Andeliana David de Sousa Rodrigues[2],
Allan de Jesus Reis Albuquerque[3] and Sandra Aparecida Marinho[1]

*Address all correspondence to: andreacbsilva@gmail.com

1 Graduate Program in Dentistry, Center of Sciences, Technology and Health, State University of Paraiba, UEPB, Araruna, Paraíba, Brazil

2 Graduate Program in Dentistry, Integrated College of Patos, FIP, Patos, Paraíba, Brazil

3 Brazilian Northeast Network on Biotechnology, RENORBIO, Federal University of Paraiba, UFPB, João Pessoa, Paraíba, Brazil

References

[1] Nagler RM, Hershkovich O, Lischinsky S, Diamond, E, Reznick, AZ. Saliva analysis in the clinical setting: revisiting an underused diagnostic tool. J. Investig. Med 2002;50(3) 214–225.

[2] Aps JKM, Martens, LC. Review: the physiology of saliva and transfer of drugs into saliva. Forensic Sci. Int 2005;150(2-3) 119–131.

[3] Humphrey SP, Williamson RT. A review of saliva: normal composition, flow, and function. J. Prosthet. Dent 2001;85(2) 162-169.

[4] Leite GJ, Mamede RCM, Leite, MGJ. Medida do Fluxo Salivar: Refinamentos ao Método do Cuspe e Uso do Papel de Filtro. Rev. Brasil. Otorrinolaringol 2002;68(6) 826-832.

[5] Jenkins GN. The Physiology of the Mouth. 3rd ed. London: The Alden Press, 1970.

[6] Edgar WM. Saliva and dental health. Clinical implications of saliva: report of a consensus meeting. Br. Dent. J 1990;169(3-4) 96-98.

[7] Arnold AMD, Marek CA. The impact of saliva on patient care: A literature review. J. Prosthet. Dent 2002;88(3) 337-343.

[8] Mandel, ID. The function of saliva. J. Dent. Res 1987;66, 623-627.

[9] Slomiany BL, Murty VL, Poitrowski J, Slomiany A. Salivary mucins in oral mucosal defense. Gen Pharmacol 1996;27(5) 761-771.

[10] Tabak LA. Stucture and function of human salivary mucins. Crit. Rev. Oral Biol. Med 1990;1(4) 229-234.

[11] Koelle DM, Huang ML, Chandran B, Vieira J, Piepcorn M, Corey L. Frequent detection of Kaposi's sarcoma-associated herpesvirus (human herpesvirus 8) DNA in saliva of human immunodeficiency virus-infected man: clinical and immunologic correlates. J Infect Dis 1997;176, (1) 94-102.

[12] Reilly TG, Poxon V, Sanders DS, Elliott TS, Walt RP. Comparison of serum, salivary, and rapid whole blood diagnostic tests for *Helicobacter pylori* and their validation against endoscopy based tests. Gut, London 1997;40(4).

[13] Giannobile WV, Beikler T, Kinney JS, Ramseier CA, Morelli T, Wong DT. Saliva as a diagnostic tool for periodontal disease: current state and future directions. Periodontology 2000;50, 52-64. DOI: 10.1111/j.1600-0757.2008.00288.x.

[14] Keyes, PH. The infectious and transmissible nature of experimental dental caries. Arch. Oral Biol 1960;1, 304-320. Doi: 10.1016/0003-9969(60)90091-1.

[15] Pihlstrom BL, Michalowicz BS, Johnson NW. Periodontal diseases 2005; Lancet 366(9499) 1809-1820.

[16] Mittal S, Bansal V, Garg S, Atreja G, Bansal S. The diagnostic role of Saliva—a review 2011; Journal of Clinical and Experimental Dentistry 2011;3(4) 314–320.

[17] Zhang L, Henson BS, Camargo PM, Wong DT. The clinical value of salivary biomarkers for periodontal disease 2009; Periodontol 2000;51, 25-37. Doi: 10.1111/j. 1600-0757.2009.00315.x.

[18] Bretas LP, Rocha ME, Vieira MS, Rodrigues ACP. Fluxo Salivar e Capacidade Tamponante da Saliva como Indicadores de Susceptibilidade à Doença Cárie. Pesq Bras Odontoped Clin Integr 2008;8(3) 289-293. Doi: 10.4034/1519.0501.2008.0083.0006.

[19] Bardow A, Moe D, Nyvad B, Nauntofte B. The buffer capacity and buffer systems of human whole saliva measured without loss of CO_2. Arch Oral Biol 2000;45(1) 1-12.

[20] Totan A, Greabu M, Totan C, Spinu T. Salivary aspartate aminotransferase, alanine aminotransferase and alkaline phosphatase: possible markers in periodontal diseases? Clinical Chemistry and Laboratory Medicine 2006;44(5) 612–615.

[21] Ramseier CA, Morelli T, Kinney JS, Dubois M, Rayburn LA, Giannobile WV (2008). Periodontal disease: salivary diagnostics. In: Salivary diagnostics. Wong DT, editor. Ames, IA: Wiley Blackwell, pp.156-168.

[22] Shimada M.H, Angelis L, Ciesielsky FIN, Gaetti-Jardim EC, Gaetti-Jardim JR E. Emprego de saliva na determinação do risco às doenças periodontais: aspectos microbiológicos e clínicos. Revista de Odontologia da UNESP 2008;37(2) 183-189.

[23] Lawrence HP. Salivary Markers of Systemic Disease: Noninvasive Diagnosis of Disease and Monitoring of General Health. Journal of the Canadian Dental Association 2002;68(3) 170-174.

[24] Vyse AJ, Brown DWG, Cohen BJ, Samuel R, Nokes DJ. Detection of rubella virus-specific immunoglobulin G in saliva by an amplification-based enzyme-linked immuno-

sorbent assay using monoclonal antibody to fluorescein isothiocyanate. J Clin Microbiol 1999;37(2) 391-395.

[25] Oliveira SA, Siqueira MM, Brown DWG, LITTON P, CAMACHO LAB, Castro ST, Cohen BJ. Diagnosis of rubella infection by detecting specific immunoglobulin M antibodies in saliva samples: a clinicbased study in Niterói, RJ, Brazil. Rev Soc Bras Med Trop 2000;33(4) 335-339.

[26] Mbulaiteye SM, Walters M, Engels EA, Bakaki PM, Ndugwa CM, Owor AM et al. High levels of Epstein-Barr virus DNA in saliva and peripheral blood from Ugandan mother-child pairs. J Infect Dis 2006;193(3) 422-426.

[27] Baron S. Oral transmission of HIV, a rarity: emerging hypotheses. J Dent Res 2001;80(7) 1602-1604.

[28] Malamud, D. Saliva as a diagnostic fluid. BMJ, London 1992;305(6847) 207-208.

[29] Malamud D. Oral diagnostic testing for detecting human immunodeficiency virus-1 antibodies: a technology whose time has come. Am J Med 1997;102(4A) 9-14.

[30] Shugars DC, Slade GD, Patton LL, Fiscus SA. Oral and systemic factors associated with increased levels of human immunodeficiency virus type 1 RNA in saliva. Oral Surg Oral Med Oral Pathol Oral Radiol Endod 2000;89(4) 432-40.

[31] Greabu M, Battino M, Mohora M et al., Saliva—a diagnostic window to the body, both in health and in disease. Journal of Medicine and Life 2009;2(2), 124–132.

[32] Malamud D. Saliva as a diagnostic fluid. Dental Clinics of North America 2011;55(1) 159–178.

[33] Ahmadi Motamayel F, Davoodi P, Dalband, M, Hendi SS. Saliva as a mirror of the body health. DJH Journal 2010;1(2), 1–15.

[34] Bhoola KD, McNicol MW, Oliver S, Foran J. Changes in salivary enzymes in patients with sarcoidosis. The New England Journal of Medicine 1969;281(16) 877–879.

[35] Bradley K, Formaker BK, Frank ME. Taste function in patients with oral burning. Chem Senses 2000;25(5), 575-81.

[36] Hershkovich O, Nagler RM. Biochemical analysis of saliva and taste acuity evaluation in patients with burning mouth syndrome, xerostomia and/or gustatory disturbances. Arch Oral Biol 2004;49(7) 515-22.

[37] Nater UM. et al. Human salivary alpha-amilase reactivity in a psychosocial stress paradigm. Int J Psychophysiol 2005;55(3) 333-342.

[38] Kristenson M, Garvin P, Lundberg U, editors. The role of saliva cortisol measurement in health and disease. EAE: Bentham Science Publishers; 2012.

[39] Naumova, E.A., Sandulescu, T., Bochnig, C., Al Khatib, Lee WK, Zimmer S, Arnold WH. Dynamic changes in saliva after acute mental stress. Scientific Reports 2014;4, 1-9. Doi: 10.1038/srep04884.

[40] Rhoades, R. A.; Tanner, G. A. Fisiologia médica. 2. Ed. Rio de Janeiro: Guanabara-Koogan, 741p, 2005.

[41] Nierop, A. et al. Prolonged salivary cortisol recovery in second-trimester pregnant women and attenuated salivary α-amylase responses to psychosocial stress in human pregnancy. J Clin Endocrinol Metab 2006;91(4), 1329-35.

[42] Kang, Y. Psychological stress-induced chances in salivary alpha-amylase and adrenergic activity. Nurs Health Sci 2010;12(4), 477-484.

[43] Savage NW, Seymour, GJ, Kruger, B.J. T-lymphocyte subset changes in recurrent aphthous stomatitis. Oral Surg Oral Med Oral Pathol 1985;60(2) 175-181.

[44] Buño, IJ. et al. Elevated levels of interferon gamma, tumor necrosis factor α, interleukins 2, 4 and 5, but not interleukin 10, are present in recurrent aphthous stomatitis. Arch Dermatol 1999;134(7) 827-831.

[45] Volkov, I. et al. Case Report: Recurrent aphthous stomatitis responds to vitamin B12 treatment. Can Fam Physician 2005;51(6) 844-845.

[46] Jurge S. et al. Recurrent aphthous stomatitis. Oral Dis 2006;12(1) 1-21.

[47] Chavan M. et al. Recurrent aphthous stomatitis: a review. J Oral Pathol Med 2012;41(8) 577-583.

[48] Lamm ME, Nedrud JG, Kaetzel CS, Mazanec MB. IgA and mucosal defense. APMIS - Acta Pathol Microbiol Immunol Scand 1995;103(4) 241-6.

[49] Truedsson L, Baskin B, Pan Q, Rabbani H, Vorechovsky I, Smith CI. Genetics of IgA deficiency. Acta Pathol Microbiol Immunol Scand 1995;103(12) 833-72.

[50] Kilian M, Reinholdt J, Lomholt T, Poulsen K, Frandsen EV. Biological significance of IgA1 proteases in bacterial colonization and pathogenesis: critical evaluation of experimental evidence. APMIS - Acta Pathol Microbiol Immunol Scand 1996;104(5) 321-38.

[51] Hucklebridge F, Lambert S, Clow A, Warburton DM, Evans PD, Sherwood N. Modulation of secretory immunoglobulin A in saliva; response to manipulation of mood. Biol Psychol 2000;53(1) 25-35.

[52] Kamodyová N, Durdiaková J, Celec P, Sedláčková T, Repiská G, Sviežená B, Minárik G. Prevalence and persistence of male DNA identified in mixed saliva samples after intense kissing. Forensic Sci Int Genet 2013;7(1) 124-8.

[53] Vieira LAC, Feijó GCS, Zara LF, Castro, CFS, Bezerra ACB. Atomic Spectroscopy Identifies Differences in Trace Element Parameters in theSaliva of Patients with Cystic Fibrosis. Pesq Bras Odontoped Clin Integr 2011;11(2) 211-216.

[54] Fabian TK, Fejerdy P, Csermely, P. Salivary Genomics, Transcriptomics and Proteomics: The Emerging Concept of the Oral Ecosystem and their Use in the Early Diagnosis of Cancer and other Diseases. Curr Genomics 2008;9(1) 11-21.

[55] Streckfus C et al., The presence of soluble cerbB-2 concentrations in the saliva and serum among women with breast carcinoma: a preliminary study. Clin Cancer Res 2000;6(6) 2363-2370.

[56] Streckfus C et al., Reliability assessment of soluble c-erbB-2 concentrations in the saliva of healthy women and men. Oral Surg Oral Med Oral Pathol Oral Radiol Endod 2001;91(2) 174-179.

[57] Bigler LR. et al. The potential use of saliva to detect recurrence of disease in women with breast carcinoma. J Oral Pathol Med 2002;31(7) 421-431.

[58] Franzmann EJ et al. Salivary soluble CD44: a potential molecular marker for head and neck cancer. Cancer Epidemiol Biomarkers Prev 2005;14(3) 735-739.

[59] Pai SI, Westra WH. Molecular pathology of head and neck cancer: implications for diagnosis, prognosis, and treatment. Annu Rev Pathol 2009;4(49) 70.

[60] Jiang WW et al., Increased mitochondrial DNA content in saliva associated with head and neck cancer. Clin Cancer Res 2005;11(7) 2486-2491. 2005.

[61] Arellano-Garcia ME et al., Multiplexed immunobead-based assay for detection of oral cancer protein biomarkers in saliva. Oral Dis 2008;14(8) 705-712.

[62] HU S, LOO JA, WONG DT. Human body fluid proteome analysis. Proteomics 2006;6(23) 6326-6353.

[63] Hu S, Loo JA, Wong DT. Human saliva proteome analysis and disease biomarker discovery. Expert Rev Proteomics 2007;4(4) 531-538.

[64] Silva RHA et al., Human bite identification and DNA technology in forensic dentistry. Brazilian Journal Oral Science 2006;19(5) 1193-1197.

[65] FARAH, S.B. DNA: segredos & mistérios. São Paulo: Sarvier; 1997.

[66] Burger J et al,. DNA preservation: a microsatellite-DNA study on ancient skeletal remains. Eletrophoresis 1999;20(8) 1722-1728.

[67] Nq, DP, Koh D, Choo SG, Ng V, Fu Q. Effect of storage conditions on the straction of PCR-quality genomic DNA from saliva. Clinica Chimica Acta 2004;343(1-2) 191-194, 2004.

[68] Ghafouri B. et al. Mapping of proteins in human saliva using two-dimensional gel electrophoresis and peptide mass fingerprinting. Proteomics 2003;3(6) 1003 -1015.

[69] TZ, C., F. et al. Complexity of the human whole saliva proteome. Physiol. Biochem 2005; 61(3) 469–480.

[70] Hirtz C et al. MS characterization of multiple forms of alpha-amylase in human saliva. Proteomics 2005;5(17) 4597-607.

[71] Messana I, Cabras T, Inzitari R, et al. Characterization of the human salivary basic proline-rich protein complex by a proteomic approach. J Proteome Res 2004;3(4) 792-800.

[72] Xie H et al., A Catalogue of Human Saliva Proteins Identified by Free Flow Electrophoresis-based Peptide Separation and Tandem Mass Spectrometry. Proteomics 2005;4(11) 1826–1830.

[73] Fridez F, Coquoz R. PCR DNA typing of stamps: evaluation of the DNA extraction. Forensic Sci Int 1996;78(2) 103–110.

[74] Barni F, Berti A, Rapone CB, Lago G. a-Amylase Kinetic Test in Bodily Single and Mixed Stains. Journal of Forensic Science 2006;51(6) 1389-1396.

[75] Wong DT. Salivary diagnostics powered by nanotechnologies, proteomics and genomics. JADA 2006;137(3) 313-321.

[76] Bonne NJ, Wong DTW. Salivary biomarker development using genomic, proteomic and metabolomic approaches. Genome Medicine 2012;4(82) 1-12.

[77] Ramachandran P, Boontheung P, Xie Y, Sondej M, Wong DT, Loo JA. Identification of Nlinked glycoproteins in human saliva by glycoprotein capture and mass spectrometry. JProteome Res 2006;5(6) 1493-1503.

[78] Nunes AP, Oliveira IO, Santos BR, Millech C, Silva LP, Gonzalez DA, Hallal PC, Menezes AM, Araujo CL, Barros FC. Quality of DNA extracted from saliva samples collected with the Oragene DNA self-collection kit. BMC Med Res Methodol 2012.

[79] Park NJ, Zhou H, Elashoff D, Henson BS, Kastratovic DA, Abemayor E, Wong DT. Salivary microRNA: discovery, characterization, and clinical utility for oral cancer detection. Clin Cancer Res 2009;15(17) 5473-5477.

[80] Garcia JM, Garcia V, Pena C, Dominguez G, Silva J, Diaz R, Espinosa P, Citores MJ, Collado M, Bonilla F. Extracellular plasma RNA from colon cancer patients is confined in a vesicle-like structure and is mRNA-enriched. RNA 2008;14(7) 1424-1432.

[81] Tinzl M, Marberger M, Horvath S, Chypre C. DD3 RNA analysis in urine? A new perspective for detecting prostate cancer. Eur Urol 2004;46(2) 182-187.

[82] Kumar SV, Hurteau GJ, Spivack SD. Validity of messenger RNA expression analyses of human saliva. Clin Cancer Res 2006;12(17) 5033-5039.

[83] Lee YH, Zhou H, Reiss JK, Yan X, Zhang L, Chia D, Wong DT. Direct saliva transcriptome analysis. Clin Chem 2011;57(9) 1295-1302.

[84] Park NJ, Yu T, Nabili V, Brinkman BM, Henry S, Wang J, Wong DT. RNA protect sal-iva. An optimal room-temperature stabilization reagent for the salivary transcrip-tome. Clin Chem 2006;52(12) 2303-2304.

[85] Hu Z, Zimmermann BG, Zhou H, Wang J, Henson BS, Yu W, Elashoff D, Krupp G, Wong DT. Exon-level expression profiling: a comprehensive transcriptome analysis of oral fluids. Clin Chem 2008;54(5) 824-832.

[86] Liu J, Duan Y. Saliva: A potential media for disease diagnostics and monitoring. Oral Oncol 2012;48(7) 569-577.

[87] Lee A, Ghaname CB, Braun TM, Sugai JV, Teles RP, Loesche WJ, Kornman KS, Gian-nobile WV, Kinney JS. Bacterial and salivary biomarkers predict the gingival inflam-matory profile. J Periodontol 2012;83(1) 79-89.

[88] Spielmann N, Wong DT. Saliva: diagnostics and therapeutic perspectives. Oral Dis 2011;17(4) 345-354.

[89] Sugimoto M, Wong DT, Hirayama A, Soga T, Tomita M. Capillary electrophoresis mass spectrometry-based saliva metabolomics identified oral, breast and pancreatic cancer-specific profiles. Metabolomics 2010;6(1) 78-95.

[90] Wei J, Xie G, Zhou Z, Shi P, Qiu Y, Zheng X, Chen T, Su M, Zhao A, Jia W. Salivary metabolite signatures of oral cancer and leukoplakia. Int J Cancer 2011;129(9) 2207-2217.

[91] Li X, Yang T, Lin J. Spectral analysis of human saliva for detection of lung cancer us-ing surface-enhanced Raman spectroscopy. J Biomed Opt 2012;17(037003).

8

Fränkel Functional Regulator in Early Treatment of Skeletal Distal and Mesial Bite

Zorana Stamenković and Vanja Raičković

1. Introduction

Skeletal distal and mesial bite are irregularities in sagittal direction. During treatment of these malocclusions we want to achieve correct occlusion and morphology, right implementation of all orofacial functions and good facial aesthetics. If we start with orthodontic treatment in early mixed dentition we can expect good and stabile therapeutic results and we can prevent later developmental problems. This way, we avoid treatment with fixed appliances in permanent dentition and orthognatic surgery after the end of growth. It is important given the fact that orthodontic treatment is very expensive.

Etiology of skeletal distal and mesial bite are heredity and some exogenous etiologic factors. These malocclusions are inherited polygenically. Skeletal distal bite is often present among the members of the same family and among twins. Other general etiological factors are Pierre Robin syndrome, syndrome of hemifacial microsomia and endocrine disorders. Local etiological factors, are, mostly, bad habits, in the age after the third year of life. The most important bad habit is thumb sucking, which causes protrusion of the upper and retrusion of the lower incisors and increasing of overjet. Skelatal distal bite is one of symptoms in CMD, as a result of ankylosis and trauma of TMJ. Dodic [1] found that 79.9% patients with skeletal class II has positive index of CMD. Etiology of skeletal mesial bite are heredity, some specific factors, functional effects, trauma and environmental factors [2]. Previously it was thought that this malocclusion was inherited as an autosomal dominant trait. Accordingly there is the existence of the so-called Habsburgs mandible. Many members of the Habsburg monarchy had a typical large lower jaw and skeletal mesial bite [3]. If in a family exists severe skeletal Class III in 33% of their children will appear Class III and in 17% of their siblings. Some scientific studies find that there is a gene which is related to mandibular prognathism. There is different expressivity of genes in specific types of progeny. Different genetic locus are responsible for the definitive form of the lower jaw. Other local etiologic factors are enlarged tonsils, breathing through the mouth and early extraction of deciduous molars. Patients with cleft lip and palate and some syndromes (Apert, Crouzon) often have mesial bite due to insufficient growth of the upper jaw.

Skeletal distal bite is most common in white population (38%), two times more frequent than in members of black race(20%), while frequency of this malloclusion in yellow race is 10-15%. The frequency of skeletal distal bite decreases with age, from 25-30% in mixed dentition, 20-25% in early permanent dentition to 15-20% in adult population [4]. Mesial bite commonly occurs among members of the yellow race with a frequency of 4% to 14% because they have underdeveloped nasomaxillary complex and deficient growth of the upper jaw. In the black population frequency of mesial bite is between 5% and 8%, while in the white population frequency of this malocclusion is from 1% to 4%. Frequency of malocclusion increases during the time. Skeletal mesial bite occurs in 23% in deciduous dentition, 30% in mixed dentition and 34% in permanent dentition.

2. Aim

The aim of this investigation was to compare clinical effects of different mobile orthodontic appliances (active and functional) in early treatment of skeletal distal (Class II division 1) and mesial (pseudo Class III) bite.

3. Material and method

In this study 60 patients were included with skeletal distal bite caused by mandibular retrognatism. All patients with this malocclusion had increasing value of angle ANB (>4°), due to the decrease of angle SNB (<80°). Main clinical characteristics of skeletal distal bite caused by mandibular retrognatism are: convexity of facial profile with distal position of the lower lip and chin and protrusion of the upper lip, distal relationship of dental arch and jaw bases, protrusion of the upper incisors and retrusion of the lower incisors with increasing value of overjet, inserting of the lower lip between upper and lower incisors, passing of the upper and lower incisors during eruption and their supraposition, traumatic deep bite, short mandibular corpus and lower dental arch, narrow and elongated upper dental arch, expressed mentolabial and nasolabial sulcus, shortened lower third of face and retroinclination of the lower jaw. Clinical effects were analysed on 60 patients with skeletal distal bite, without earlier orthodontic treatment. Patients were divided in three groups, with 20 patients in each. First group was treated with FR-I, second with bionator by Balters type I and the third group with Hotz mobile appliance. Effects were determined on study casts and lateral cephalometrics before and after treatment, and during functional clinical examinations and analysis of facial aesthetics.

Also, in this study were included 40 patients with skeletal Class III caused by maxillary retrognatism. They have typical changes in facial aesthetic and profile. All patients had decreasing value of angle ANB (<2°), due do decrease of angle SNA (<82°). Main clinical characteristics of pseudo Class III (caused by maxillary retrognatism) are: concavity of the facial profile with distal position of the upper lip and correct position of the lower lip and chin, mesial relationship of dental arches and jaw bases, normoinclination of upper and lower incisors, narrow and short upper dental arch, reverse overjet, lateral cross bite, underdeveloped nasomaxillary complex, crowding in upper dental arch, anteinclination of the upper jaw and changes in vertical direction. In this group of patients, also, study casts and profile teleradiograms have been analysed before and after orthodontic treatment.

Growth modification is possible if we start with orthodontic treatment early enough, before pubertal growth acceleration. Ideal period for growth modification is early mixed dentition. In this period we can affect the size and position of upper and lower jaw and their relationship. In girls treatment should be initiated at an earlier age than in boys, approximately two years. In girls "juvenile acceleration" starts 1-2 years before pubertal growth acceleration. Overall growth is affected by age, constitution, seasonal and cultural factors. Before orthodontic treatment it is necessary to determine skeletal maturity of our patients [5]. Treatment with growth modification is possible when patient is in one of three first stage of skeletal maturation (Fig. 1).

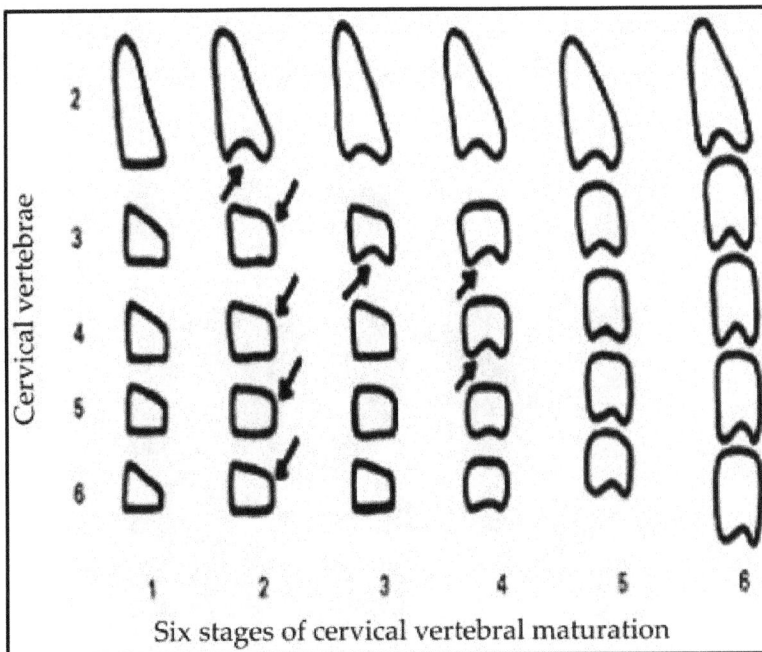

Figure 1. Six stages of cervical vertebral maturation (O'Relly & Yanneillo, 1988).

When we make decisions about growth modification treatment we need to know the degree of discrepancy between viscerocranium and neurocranium, age and sex of the patient, external and internal motivation, which appliances we want to use, at what stage of skeletal maturation is patient and how much growth left to the end of maturity [6, 7].

4. Treatment of skeletal distal bite

In modern orthodontics treatment of skeletal distal bite can be performed using many dental worn functional appliances, such as activator, bionator by Balters, twin block, Herbst appliance, Hotz appliance and vestibular plate. These appliances rest on teeth and they stimulate growth of the lower jaw due to changes in activity of orofacial muscles.

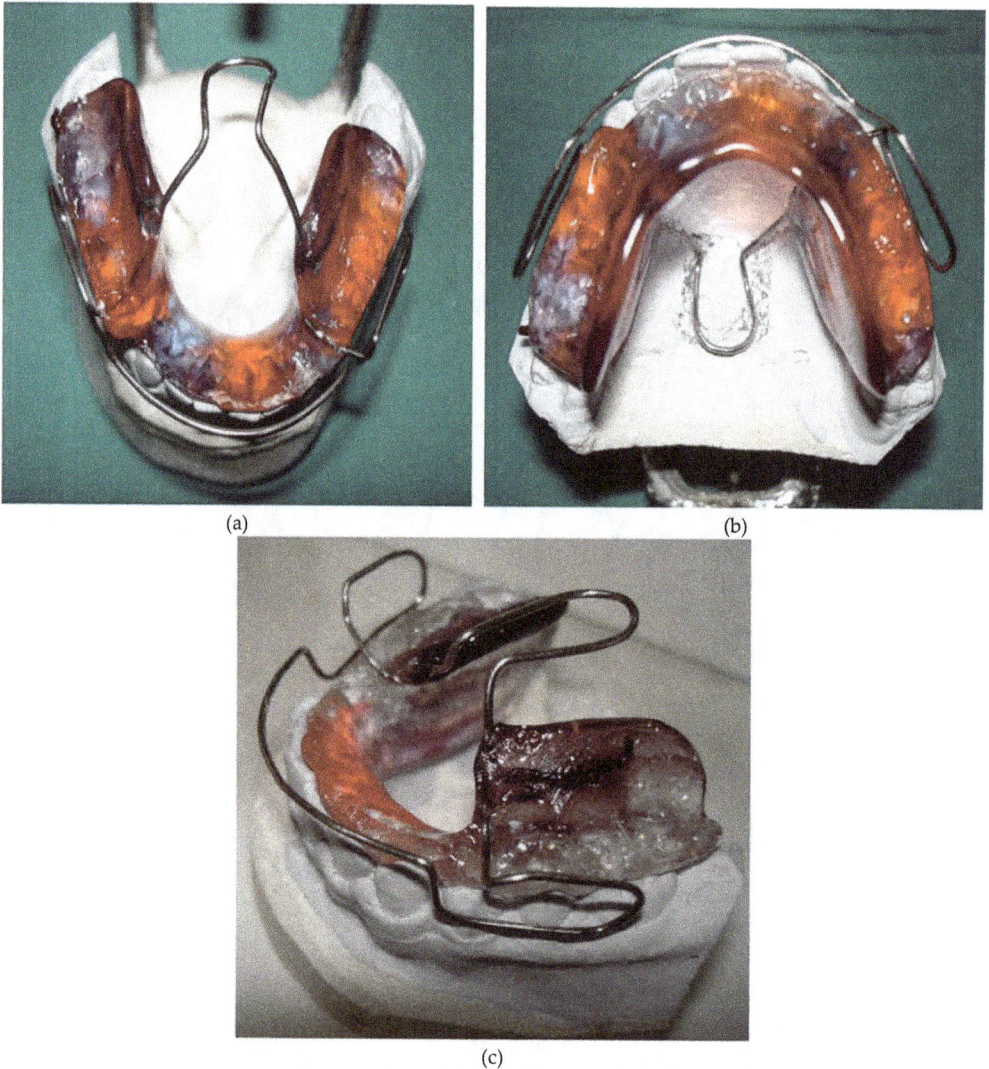

Figure 2. a.,b.,c. Balters bionator type I

To Balters opinion disturbed function, size and tone of tongue are the main cause of all malocclusions. Bionator was designed and used in orthodontic practice by Balters in Germany (1950.). Bionator by Balters type I or the standard form is used in treatment of skeletal distal bite. This appliance is known in literature as reduced activator with interoclusal acrylic.

Components of this appliance are palatal arch directed pharyngeal, vestibular arch above upper incisors and buccal loops in the area of canines (Fig 2.a.,2.b.,2.c.). Construction bite is determined and taken in incisal relationship of incisors without activation in vertical direction. Skeletal effects are increasing of mandibular corpus and ramus, anterior displacement of the lower jaw, increasing value of angle SNB and decreasing value of angle ANB [8, 9, 10].

Hotz appliance is modified active mobile orthodontic appliance. This appliance in orthodontic practice was introduced by Hotz (1966.) in Germany. Appliance has angular frontal bite plane (Fig.3.). This appliance causes growth modification and anterior growth of the lower jaw in patients with forward facial rotation. It is necessary that inclined frontal bite plane has sufficient length for anterior movement and sliding of the lower jaw [11]. Skeletal effects are stimulation of saggital growth of the lower jaw and anterior displacement. Dental effects are retrusion of the upper and protrusion of the lower incisors and extrusion of the posterior teeth [12].

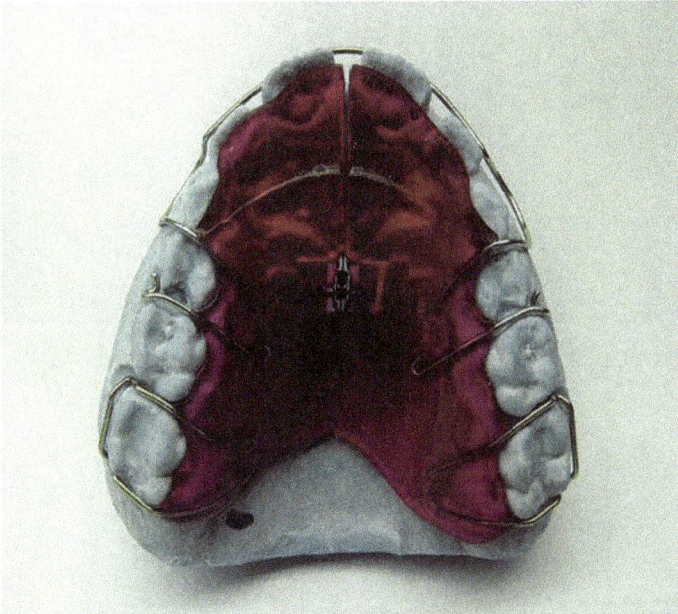

Figure 3. Hotz appliance

5. Fränkel appliance type I (FR-I)

Fränkel functional regulator (FR) is only mounted functional appliance which can effectively correct morphological (skeletal and dental) and functional irregularities. It works by pressure application at skeletal and dental structures, elimination of the pressure surrounding perioral musculature and causing tensile stress in the area of mucosal fornix, where exist bone apposition. Construction of this appliance was suggested by Rölf Fränkel in Germany (1966.)

[13]. During time the position of the lower jaw permanently changed without affecting the position of the teeth. The essential changes are tissue changes at the articular zone of growth. This appliance significantly changed muscles activity and whole physiological state of orofacial complex. There are early and late treatment of skeletal distal bite using FR-I. Early treatment begins in the age of 7-8 years, in early mixed dentition, after eruption of first permanent molars and incisors. Late treatmen starts in the age of 12 years (average) after eruption of canines and premolars [14]. Whole treatment contains active and retention period. Active period lasts an average of 18 to 24 months. During this period patient wears appliance continuously during the day, except during meals. Retention period lasts, also, 24 months. During this period patient wears appliance only at night. After 6 months of treatment sagittal relationship was corrected for half a molar width.

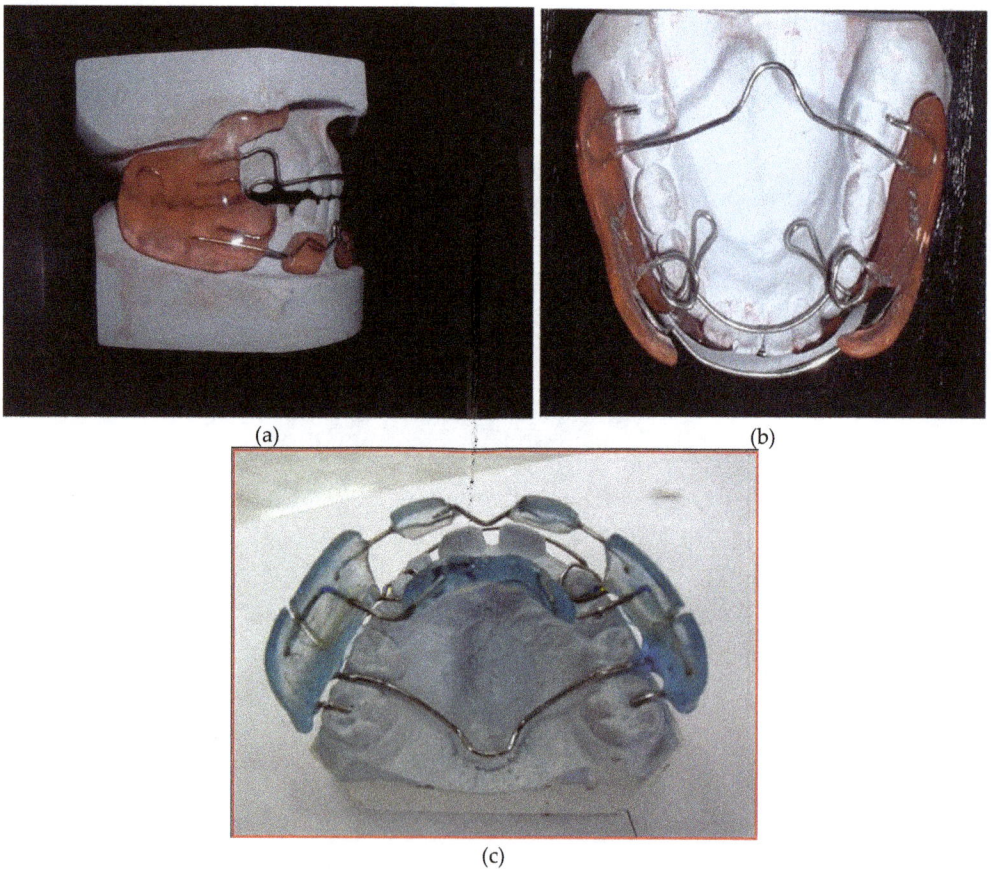

(a)   (b)

(c)

Figure 4. a.,b.,c. Fränkel appliance type I (FR-I)

In treatment of skeletal Class II we use three type of FR-I (Ia, Ib, Ic). FR-Ia is indicated for use in cases with: skeletal Class I with deep bite, skeletal Class I with protrusion of the upper and retrusion of the lower incisors, skeletal Class I with apical crowding, bilateral crossbite, skeletal Class II division 1 with overjet less than 5mm, skeletal Class II divison 1 with deep bite and retrusion of the lower incisors. FR-Ib is indicated in patients with skelelat Class II divison 1 and overjet between 5mm and 7mm and skeletal Class II divison 1. with deep bite. FR-Ic is indicated for use in cases with severe skeletal Class II divison 1 and overjet over 7mm, skeletal Class II with deep bite and difficulties to establish contact between lips during anterior movement of the lower jaw. Components of this appliance (FR-Ia) are: lateral acrilyc shields, pelotas for lower lip, labial arch, linqual arch, palatal arch with anchorage on the upper first molars and loops for upper canines (Fig. 4a.,b.,c.). For construction and making of this appliance is necessary construction bite in incisal relation of incisors without activation in vertical direction (Fig.5.). FR-Ib besides these elements includes linqual shield with linqual arch and additional arch for protrusion of the lower incisors. For FR-Ic we determine and take construction bite in relation of Class I on posterior teeth. This appliance has screw for compensatory anterior movement of the lower jaw. Construction and design of this appliance is very gentle, so patients should be very careful during manipulation with it [15].

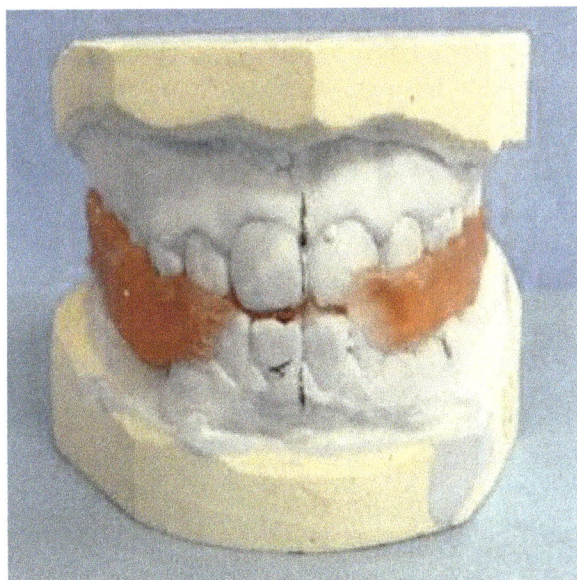

Figure 5. Construction bite for FR-I

6. Treatment of skeletal Class III

Skeletal Class III can be treated by many different dental worn functional appliances. Representatives of this group of appliances are activator, bionator by Balters type III, orthopedic bionator, chin cup, Y appliance, appliance with Bertoni screw and facial mask. The only representative of tissue worn appliances is FR-III. In older age surgical treatment is indicated in combination with fixed appliances [16].

Clinical effects were determined on 40 patients with skeletal Class III caused by maxillary retrognatism (angle SNA<82°, angle ANB<2°). None of the patients have previously had an orthodontic treatment, all of them were in period of early mixed dentition, after eruption of first permanent molars. These patients were divided in two groups, with 20 patients in each. Patients in the first group were treated by FR-III, while patients in the second group were treated by Y appliance. Clinical effects were analyzed on study casts, lateral cephalometric and facial aesthetic before and after treatment. Separately were analyzed and interpreted parameters of position and development of the upper and lower jaw, parameters of intermaxillary relations, parameters of the facial growth, the cranial base parameters, parameters of the position of the incisors, parameters of TMJ, soft tissue profile parameters, parameters of skeletal and dental changes during the treatment and methods of investigation of orofacial functions.

Y appliance is active, mobile orthodontic appliance. This appliance has acrylic plate cut to shape letter Y with two screws in the area of canine (Fig.6.). Patients turn both screws in the same time, that way the appliance causes protrusion of the upper incisors. Y appliance is useful in patients with pseudo Class III [12]. With this appliance we correct reverse overjet and eliminate premature contact with stabile treatment result. Ideal time for treatment is period of mixed dentition. Patients turn screws once in 7 days, with biological movement less than 1mm during one month. During retention period patient wear appliance only during the night, without turning the screws.

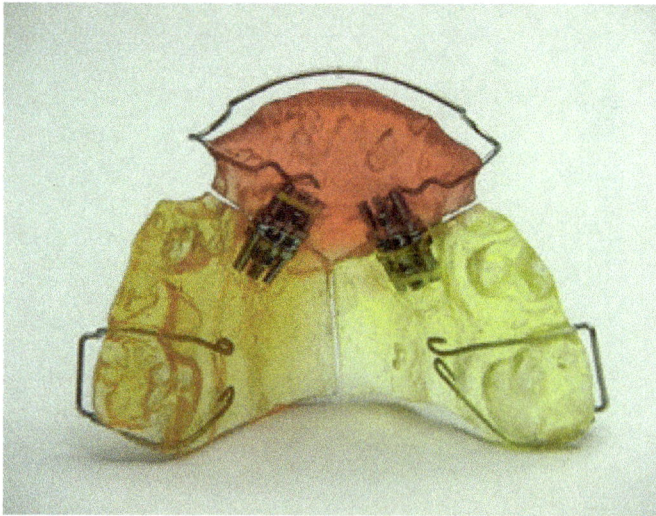

Figure 6. Y appliance

7. Fränkel appliance type III — (FR-III)

Fränkel functional regulator (FR) is passive, mobile functional appliance. At the same time it is the only tissue worn functional appliance. With FR we can correct both occlusal (dental and skeletal) and functional irregularities. Three main mechanisms of action of this device are: aplication of pressure, elimination of pressure and application of pulling force. Rölf Fränkel presented this appliance to orthodontic public in Germany in 1966. Application of pressure prevents excessive growth of the lower jaw in sagittal direction. Elimination of pressure separates the soft tissues of the lips and cheeks and prevents their contact with dentoalveolar structures. FR-III contributes to the proper formation of dentoalveolar structures of the upper and lower jaw. Application of pulling force increases the activity of osteoblasts in the periost, that way appliance contributes to the creation of new bone tissue in the upper jaw [17]. Acrylic pelotas are located in the upper vestibule and stimulate the sagittal growth of the upper jaw. FR-III causes tissue changes in the articular zone of growth. During wearing of appliance there is a continual activation of the muscles of the orofacial region to change their tone and activity. Optimal time for treatment with this appliance is early mixed dentition, immediately after eruption of all upper permanent molars, at an age of about seven years of age. The best therapeutic results are expected in patients with reverse overjet (4-5mm). The whole therapeutic procedure contains active and retention phase. Active phase lasts 24 to 30 months. During this active period, patients wear FR-III continuosly during the day and night, except during meals. Retention phase lasts about 24 months. During retention period, patients wear appliance only at night. This phase is important to preserve the stabile therapeutic results. From this we can conclude that the total duration of therapy is quite long. Patients can easily get used to this appliance, it is comfortable to use, they are motivated for treatment and we expect full cooperation with them and their parents. In treatment of skeletal Class III we use Fränkel functional regulator type III (FR-III). There are two different types, type FR-IIIa and type FR-IIIb. Type FR-IIIa is indicated in early mixed dentition in patients with pseudo mesial byte and deep reverse overjet. Type FR-IIIb is indicated in early mixed dentition in patients with pseudo mesial byte, but without deep reverse overjet. Contraindications for treatment with FR-III are: late age of patients, skeletal Class III caused by mandibular prognatism, severe teeth rotation and malpositions and coronary crowding. FR-IIIa consists of: two lateral vestibular acrylic shields, pelotas for upper lip, lower labial arch, bilatteral posterior acrylic plate on teeth, wire anchorage on the lower first permanent molars, palatal arch with protrusion arch in the upper jaw and wire elements between pelotas and shileds (Fig. 7a.,b.,c.). FR-IIIb has simillar construction. The only difference is that FR-III does not have bilatteral posterior acrylic plate on teeth, because it is indicated in cases without deep reverse overjet, and in this situation desarticulation is not necessary. Construction and design of this appliance are very delicate. That is why patients must be very careful and patient during wearing and manipulation with FR-III. The most important phase in the development of this device is taking an accurate construction bite. Construction bite determines the position of the lower jaw in all directions. For this appliance construction bite is taken in maximal retrusion of the lower jaw, with proper midline alignment of the upper and lower jaw. The ideal would be to provide edge to edge contacts between upper and lower incisors in sagittal direction. Activation in vertical direction depends of depth of reverse overjet. In cases with deep reverse overjet, construction bite is taken with vertical activation of 2-4mm above the physiologic rest position. If patients do not have deep reverse overjet, construction bite is taken without activation in vertical direction, at physiologic rest position. Design of appliance enables correct teeth eruption with elimination of irregular muscle activity. It is said that appliance causes oral gymnastics. Pelotas stimulate growth of the upper jaw and cause increase of the width of apical base. Pelotas have triple effect: elimination of the pressure of the upper lip to the sagittal underdeveloped upper jaw, creating tensile stress in the vestibule and stimulate osteoblasts activity at the level of the periost and directing the force of the upper lip to the lower jaw over the lower vestibular arch, thus resulting in retrusion Acrylic lateral shields are in contact with lower teeth and apical base, while settle 3mm of dentoalveolar structures of the upper jaw. Appliance then stimulates both, transversal and sagittal growth of underdevolped maxilla. Fränkel suggests that functional disorder is result of malocclusion, and rarely is the primary cause of the irregularities. Appliance stimulates proper orofacial functions and achieves a balance between the muscles of tongue and buccal muscles. It eliminates the disturbed functions due to activation and adaptation of muscles. It is important to wear the appliance during the day because it achieves a constant muscle activity, while the activity is significantly reduced during the night. It is necessary to examine the relationship between form and function if we want a successful therapeutic result. FR-III regulates the function of swallowing due to buccal shields. These shields eliminate the pressure of buccal muscles and allow extension of dentoalveolar structures by changing the position and functions of tongue during swallowing. This provides a transition from infantile to mature swallowing. In some patients function of tongue is changed due to adaptation to the existing malocclusion, while in other groups of patients that is the primary cause of malocclusion. FR-III significantly increases anterior and posterior width in the upper and lower jaw and length of the upper dental arch. Appliance decreases buccal inclination of the upper first permanent molar. With FR-III dental arch can expand for 6mm and alveolar base for 5mm. Palatal arch allows expansion of lateral shields, gives support to appliance and contributes to transverse anchorage of appliance. Palatal arch is 0.5mm from the mucosae. Protrusion arch has function to cause protrusion of the upper frontal teeth. Active arch is in contact with palatal surfaces of upper incisors, close to incisal edge. Therefore, arch causes protrusion of incisors without influencing their vertical eruption. Pelotas have a parallelogram shape with rounded corners. Lower edge of pelotas is located deeply in the vestibule, 2.5-3mm from mucosa and 7-8mm from gingival edge. Upper edge of pelotas is 5mm from marginal gingival edge. The appliance does not rely on the posterior teeth in the upper jaw, because in that case pelotas cause distal movement of upper posterior teeth [13, 14]. Phases in treatment and creating of FR-III are: clinical examination, functional analysis, impressions of upper and lower jaw for study casts, analysis of lateral cephalograms and orthopantomograms, construction bite, preparation of study casts, definite preparation in the laboratory, giving the appliance to the patient and regular check-ups every four to six weeks. Phase of adaptation to FR-III is longer than with the other functional appliances. A common protocol is that patient wears the appliance for 2 hours a day for first two weeks of therapy. Next two weeks the appliance is worn for 4 hours a day. At the next check-up the appliance wearing time extends to 6 hours a day in combination with speech exercise. After the third control check-up, it is recommended to wear the appliance at all times for 24 hours, except during meals. After three months of properly wearing of appliance changes in sagittal, vertical and transversal direction are observed. Generally, after six months of treatment, skeletal Class III is corrected for half a premolar width. If there is lateral open bite it is a sign of good cooperation of the patient, because the changes in the vertical plane are more slowly than in the transversal and vertical direction, and eruption of the lower posterior teeth happens later.

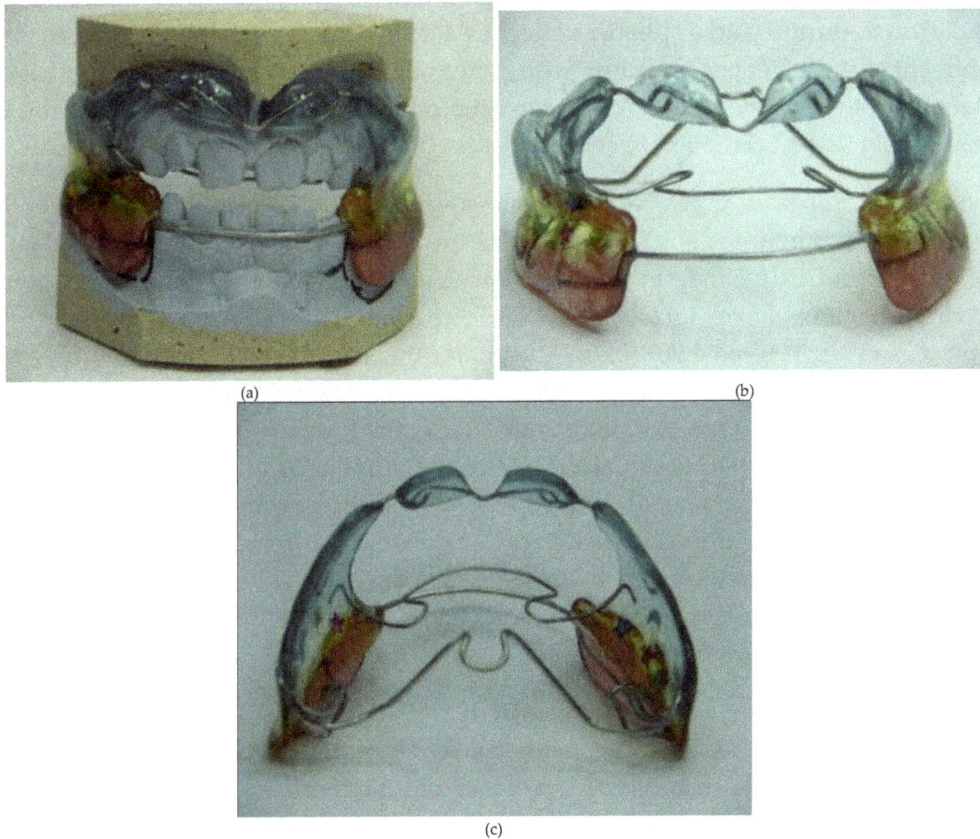

Figure 7. a.,b.,c. Fränkel appliance type III (FR-III)

8. Results and discusion

8.1. Comparative analysis of the FR-I appliance, bionator by Balters and Hotz appliance treatment effects

Position and development of the upper jaw were analyzed using values of angles SNA, SN/SpP and J and linear distance which determines length of maxillary corpus. All used appliances didn't have significant impact on position of the upper jaw. Their effects were directed to the lower jaw. Changes on the lower jaw were determined using values of angles SNB, SN/MP and SNPg and linear distances of length of mandibular corpus, total length of lower jaw, height and width of mandibular ramus. All appliances significantly changed sagittal position of the lower jaw [18]. The most pronounced increase of angle SNB causes FR-

I from 74.70° to 77.65° (p=0.001*). FR-I and bionator by Balters type I cause reducing of vertical inclination of the lower jaw to the anterior cranial base, while Hotz appliance causes increasing of vertical inclination of the lower jaw. Analysis of linear parameters showed mandibular growth in all directions, especially during the application of FR-I. Length of mandibular corpus increased from 71.22mm to 73.20mm. Malocclusion was corrected due to the joint effect of the pubertal growth process and appliances effects. All effects of appliances resulting in anterior displacement of the lower jaw and chin, with increasing value of angle SNB, without affecting the total amount of growth. In some cases existed inhibition of sagittal growth of the upper jaw, resulting in better relation between jaw bases [19, 20, 21].

Interjaw relationship was analyzed using values of angles ANB (sagittal interjaw angle), B (basal angle-vertical interjaw angle), SpP/OcCP (inclination between upper jaw and occlusal plane) and MP/OcCP (inclination between lower jaw and occlusal plane). All appliances caused the correction of skeletal Class II with decreasing values of ANB angle from 6.60° to 3.60° (p<0.001 FR-I), 5.90° na 4.90° (p=0.001 bionator by Balters type I), 5.80° to 5.10° (p=0.032 Hotz appliance). Skeletal effect was greater in the younger age. After that age, in permanent dentition, dental effects were dominant. FR-I changed function and activity of orofacial muscles and caused their transformation [22].When appliance is in the mouth vestibular pelotas provide anterior movement of the lower jaw. "U" loop prevents distal movement of the lower jaw in initial position. It is necessary to provide at the same time growth stimulation of the lower jaw and adaptation of soft tissues. This is the only way therapeutic result can be stabile and long-term. It is suggested to provide neutroocclusion through several phases, with gradually mesial movement of the lower jaw, using construction bite.

FR-I decreased basal angle, while bionator by Balters type I and Hotz appliance (p=0.044) increased value of this angle. These appliances are contraindicated in patients with backward facial rotation, because the use of this appliance would result in opening of the bite and divergent growth of jaw bases [23]. All used appliances increased vertical inclination of the upper jaw to the occlusal plane, without statistical significance. FR-I indicated anteinclination of the lower jaw to the occlusal plane, while Hotz appliance and bionator by Balters type I caused retroinclination of the lower jaw. Hotz appliance caused extrusion of posterior teeth, which reduced overbite and contributed to the opening of the bite. These changes are consequence of movement of fossa glenoidalis during growth.

All used appliances increased values of angles NSAr and ArGoMe, while FR-I and Hotz appliance increased value of angle SArGo, but bionator by Balters type I decreased value of this angle. Sum of angles of Björk polygon were increased, most evident when using FR-I, from 393.55° to 395.70°. Mostly, patients in this sample had forward rotation before beginning of the orthodontic treatment. It was good prognostic sign for patients with skeletal Class II, while vertical growth was not significant in cases with mandibular retrognathism. If we start with orthodontic treatment early enough (in early mixed dentition) we can change type of facial growth [24, 25]. FR-I and bionator by Balters mostly didn't change type of facial growth, while Hotz appliance caused backward rotation and vertical facial growth. During therapeutic procedure anterior and posterior facial height were decreased, partially as a consequence of intensive growth in this age and as a result of used appliances. Simillar changes were registred on both, anterior and posterior facial height, but facial growth in total was not changed during this period. Both methods, Björk and Jarabak, are metric, static and they show type of facial growth in one moment. That's why these methods are not reliable for long-term research.

Changes on the cranial base were analyzed by linear distances N-S (length of anterior cranial base), S-Ba (length of posterior cranial base) and N-Ba (total length of cranial base) and angle of cranial base NSBa. All parameters were increased during orthodontic treatment. Changes in linear distances were not statistically significant during this period. Thereby distance N-Se can be used as a reference plane for superposition of lateral cephalometrics for longitudinal studies. Changes in linear distances were primarily consequence of intensive facial growth in this period, not as a effect of used appliances [26]. Angle NSBa was increased during treatment with FR-I and Hotz appliance, while bionator by Balters type I caused decreasing value of angle NSBa. Size, form and structure of cranial base are under genetic control, with some specific characteristics of race and gender. Bones of cranial base are primarily in cartilage. After that enhondral ossification and bone formation begins. Whole cranial base was elongated due to the growth of synhondrosis. We cannot affect the cranial base the same way as the facial bones. Between bones of cranial base are immobile joints, so the whole cranial base appears as one long bone. When we plan orthodontic treatment we can not expect severe changes in morphology and size of cranial base. Present changes were result of intensive displacement and bone remodelation and growth on synhondrosis.

Inclination of upper incisors was changed during orthodontic treatment, angle I/SpP was increased in whole sample. All used appliances caused retrusion of upper incisors, the most visible during treatment with bionator by Balters type I (angle I/SpP was changed from 69.35° to 71.15°). Retrusion of upper incisors is one of the most important dental effects during orthodontic treatment with these appliances. In the beginnig of treatment lower incisors were, mostly retruded or had normoinclination. Position of lower incisors is important information when planning orthodontic treatment. Correct relation between lower incisors and bone jaw base is necessary for stabile therapeutic result [27, 28]. During orthodontic treatment all appliances caused protrusion of lower incisors with decreasing values of angle i/MP. FR-I caused change of this angle from 89.75° to 88.30°, Hotz appliance from 89.75° to 87.00°, with statistical significance p<0.001, while bionator by Balters type I decreased value of angle i/MP from 89.15° to 89.00°, without statistical significance. Balance between retrusion of the upper and protrusion of the lower incisors provides decreasing of overjet.

During orthodontic treatment changes on TMJ were made in two dimensions, the change in a height of TMJ (vertical direction) and anteroposterior position of TMJ (sagittal direction). TMJ is one of growth zones during this period. "Answer" of TMJ to orthodontic treatment is one of the most important facts for final therapeutic result. During orthodontic tretmant the height of TMJ was decreased, without statistical significance. Sagittal position of TMJ was analyzed by distance S-E. This distance was increased during orthodontic treatment, statistically significant during treatment with FR-I (from 22mm to 23mm) and bionator by Balters type I (p=0.042). These changes are consequence of used functional appliances and their effects to upper and lower jaw [29, 30].

Harmonious facial aesthetics means a balance between skeletal and dentoalveolar structures from one side and structures of soft tissue profile, from the other side. All structures of orofacial complex constitute one indivisible whole. Changes on soft tissue profile were determined using analysis of angles T and H, position of the upper and lower lip to aesthetic line and height of upper lip. Effects on soft tissue structures are necessary for stabile therapeutic result and good facial aesthetics. During period of growth changes on soft tissues are much more pronounced than on skeletal structures. Upper and lower lip and other soft tissues move down a function of time [31]. As a result of increasing values of angles SNB and SNPg changes in values of angles T and H appear. Angle T is in correlation with angle J and it was significantly decreased during treatment, from 21.60° to 17.15° with FR-I. Angle H is in correlation with angle ANB. With decreasing of angle ANB decreases the value of angle H. This angle was significantly decreased, most evident when using FR-I from 16.45° to 13.40°, p<0.001. Patients with skeletal distal bite have convex profile, with irregular position of the upper and lower lip. During orthodontic treatment upper lip had smaller distance to aesthetic line, when using FR-I from 0.77mm to 0.12mm. Lower lip had, also, smaller distance to aesthetic line, except when using Hotz appliance. During orthodontic treatment height of the upper lip was decreased, when using FR-I from 26.15mm to 25.85mm, while Hotz appliance and bionator by Balters increased height of the upper lip. Decreasing of profile convexity appears as a consequence of movement of the upper and lower lip to Ricketts aesthetic line [32, 33, 34].

Patients with Class II divison 1 often have disturbed orofacial functions, especially swallowing and speech. These patients have infantile swallowing with tongue insertion between upper and lower frontal teeth. FR-I has the greatest impact on correction of orofacial functions [35]. This appliance provides the transition from infantile to mature swallowing. Design of FR-I prevents insertion of lower lip and tongue between upper and lower incisors. It creates conditions for correct articulation of interdental consonants. FR-I causes continuous muscle activation and changes in tone and muscle activity [36, 37, 38].

Pancherz's analysis defines skeletal and dentoalveolar changes during orthodontic treatment. Measurements have been done in the area of upper and lower first permanent molars and incisors and skeletal points pg and ss [39, 40]. FR-I changed molar relation for 1.45mm, Hotz appliance for 2.12mm and bionator by Balters type I 1.15mm. Relation between incisors was changed for 2.05mm when using FR-I, 1.85mm with Hotz appliance and 1.40mm with bionator by Balters type I. Skeletal correction was the most evident when using FR-I 3.35mm, bionator by Balters type I changed it for 2.80mm and Hotz appliance for 2.40mm.

8.2. Review of clinical effects using FR-III and Y appliance in treatment of skeletal Class III

Dimensions, position and development of the upper jaw were analyzed using values of angles SNA (angle of maxillary prognatism), SN/SpP (vertical position of the upper jaw to anterior cranial base) and J (angle of facial inclination), and linear distances Cmax which determines the length of the upper jaw. Both appliances had significant effect to the upper jaw, causing her anterior movement in relation to the anterior cranial base and increase the value of the angle SNA, with statistical significance p<0.001*. FR-III caused increasing of SNA angle from 76.65° to 79.85°, while Y appliance increased this angle from 76.60° to 77.90° Both appliances caused increasing of vertical inclination of the upper jaw to the anterior cranial base. This has resulted in increasing values of angle SN/SpP, with FR-III from 10.20° to 10.50° and with Y appliance from 11.75° to 12.75°. Y appliance caused significant increasing of angle J, from 80.45° to 81.90°. FR-III, also, caused, an increase in the angle J, but to a much lesser extent, from 83.10° to 83.35°. In the whole sample there was a significant increase in the value of the upper jaw length corpus, with FR-III from 43.24mm to 46.15mm and with Y appliance from 46.87mm to 48.35mm. Increasing of maxillary corpus length is a result of simultaneously intensive growth and effect of orthodontic appliance [41, 42, 43]. Position, development and dimension of the lower jaw vere analyzed by angles SNB (angle of mandibular prognatism), SN/MP (angle of vertical position of the lower jaw to the anterior cranial base) and SNPg (sagittal position of chin to the anterior cranial base) and linear parameters: length of mandibular corpus, total length of the lower jaw, height and width of mandibular ramus. Changes in the lower jaw are low, which is in accordance with the design of the appliances, and design of the appliances, and mainly the upper jaw. FR-III increased value of angle SNB from 78.55° to 78.60°, while Y appliance increased this angle from 79.00° to 79.45°. Both appliances caused retroinclination of the lower jaw and increasing of angle SN/SpP. FR-III caused changes of SN/MP angle from 35.40° to 36.65° and Y appliance from 36.85°to 38.90°. Angle SNPg was increased during the treatment, in correlation with increasing of SNB angle. Y appliance caused major changes from 79.45° to 80.05°, while FR-III increased this angle from 78.80° to 79.30°. Appliances caused retroinclination of the lower jaw to the anterior cranial base and inhibiting the growth of the lower jaw. All linear parameters were increased, mostly as a result of facial growth. Length of mandibular corpus was increased from 68.85mm to 70.00mm using FR-III, while Y appliance caused change from 73.55mm to 74.75mm. Total length of the upper jaw was increased with FR-III from 104.05mm to 105.60mm and with Y appliance from 118.10mm to 118.55mm. FR-III increased height of mandibular ramus from 52.77mm to 53.70mm, while Y appliance changed this parameter from 54.15mm to 54.95mm. Both appliances increased width of the mandibular ramus, FR-III from 11.55mm to 12.55mm and Y appliance from 11.15mm to 12.10mm. All effects of appliances resulted in anterior movement of the upper jaw and stimulation of maxillary sagittal and transversal growth [44, 45, 46, 47].

Relationship between upper and lower jaw was determined by values of angles ANB (sagittal interjaw angle, skeletal Class), B or SpP/MP (basal angle – vertical interjaw angle), SpP/OcCP (vertical postion of the upper jaw to occlusal plane) and MP/OcCP (vertical position of the lower jaw to occlusal plane). Both appliances caused significant increasing value of ANB angle. It allows correction of skeletal Class III to skeletal Class I. FR-III changed angle ANB from -1.90° to 1.25°, while Y appliance changed this angle from -2.40° to -1.55°, with statistical significance on the level $p=0.001$*. FR-III primarily affects the skeletal structures due to pelotas which stimulate the growth of the upper jaw, increasing its length and raise the value of ANB angle. Increasing value of ANB angle is a consequence of increasing the value of the angle SNA. Mobile, active appliances mostly affect dentoalveolar structures and skeletal changes are minimal. During the treatment, both appliances increased value of basal angle (B). It can contribute to opening bite. FR-III increased value of angle B from 25.20° to 26.30° and Y appliance changed angle B from 25.05° to 26.15°. Angle SpP/MP was increased during treatment, with FR-III from 10.30° to 11.45° and with Y appliance from 10.40° to 11.55°. At the same time value of angle MP/OcCp was decreased, without statistical significance, with FR-III from 14.90° to 14.85° and with Y appliance from 14.65° to 14.60°. Changes in basal angle were mostly result of increasing angle between upper jaw and occlusal plane [48, 49]. Appliances are contraindicated in patients with backward facial rotation, because their use can contribute to the bite opening and divergent growth of the bases of upper and lower jaw.

Facial growth and rotation are determined by Björk and Jarabak method. FR-III increased angle NSAr from 122.80° to 123.87° and Y appliance from 127.35° to 128.65°. Also, both appliances increased value of gonial angle-ArGoMe, FR-III from 131.10° to 131.85° and Y appliance from 131.75° to 132.15°. FR-III increased value of articular angle-SArGo from 141.50° to 142.17°, while Y appliance decreased tih angle from 134.95° to 134.25°. As a result there is an increase in values of sum of angles of Björks polygon, with FR-III from 395.40° to 396.90° and with Y appliance from 394.05° to 395.05°. Linear distances, N-Me and S-Go, were increased during this period. This increase was a consequence of pubertal facial growth in this age and use of orthodontic appliances. Relation between anterior and posterior facial height was slightly changed, without influence to total facial growth during the treatment. Relation was changed by FR-III from 64.34% to 63.35% and with Y appliance from 63.73% to 64.30%. If we start with orthodontic treatment early enough we can change the type of facial growth. Generally, FR-III caused slight backward rotation and tendency to the vertical facial growth [50, 51, 52].

FR-III and Y appliance caused increasing of length of anterior cranial base, FR-III from 68.70mm to 69.50mm, Y appliance from 71.55mm to 72.85mm. Also, both appliances increased value of total length of cranial base, FR-III from 101.30mm to 103.85mm, Y appliance from 106.85mm to 107.45mm. FR-III caused decreasing of posterior cranial base from 44.55mm to 42.70mm, while Y appliances increased this distance from 47.25mm to 47.40mm. All changes did not have statistically significance. Both appliances caused increase of angle NSBa. Increase was significant during treatment with Y appliance, which changed this angle from 130.15° to 131.35°, with statistical significance on the level $p=0.003*$. Dimension and structure of the cranial base are genetically determined. Changes on the cranial base are not a consequence of orthodontic treatment. Usually changes are results of displacement and remodelation of bones and growth of cranial base [53]. When we plan orthodontic treatment we can not expect severe changes in structures of cranial base.

Position of the upper incisors was analyzed by angle I/SpP. Usually patients with skeletal Class III (except severe mandibular prognatism) have normoinclination of the upper incisors. Both appliances significantly changed value of angle I/Spp, FR-III from 72.70° to 70.80° and Y appliance from 71.30° to 68.70°, with significance on the level $p<0.001*$. Y appliance caused, as a mobile active appliance, major changes in dentoalveolar structures. Inclination of the lower incisors was analysed by angle i/MP. FR-III increased value of angle i/MP from 89.50° to 90.60°, with statistical significance $p<0.001*$. Y appliance had no significant effect on the change of value of the angle i/MP (from 90.15° to 90.05°). It was consequence of design of appliance, which is located only on the upper jaw. Protrusion of the upper incisors and retrusion of the lower incisors created conditions for correct overjet [54, 55].

Orthodontic treatment can change vertical position (height of TMJ) and sagittal position of TMJ. TMJ is one of the growth zone during period of puberty. For stabile therapeutic results changes on the TMJ structures are very important and their answer to applied force [56]. Both appliances did not have big influence to vertical position of TMJ. FR-III changed height of TMJ from 6.15mm to 5.75mm, while Y appliance caused change from 4.55mm to 4.60mm. S-E distance was increased during treatment, which is related to the distal movement of TMJ. Y appliance caused greater increasing of S-E distance from 21.90mm to 22.65mm, with statistical significance p=0.012*. FR-III changed S-E distance from 20.40mm to 21.25mm. All changes on TMJ structures are consequence of changes on the upper and lower jaw.

Changes on soft tissue structures were analysed by angles T and H, position of the upper and lower lip to aesthetic line and height of the upper lip. Angle T is in correlation with angle J. Changes of angle J during the treatment caused increasing value of angle T in patients with skeletal Class III. FR-III increased angle T from 7.05° to 10.50°, while Y appliance increased this angle from 8.80° to 10.70°. Angle H (Holdaway) is in positive correlation with angle ANB. Patients with skeletal Class III have angle ANB<2°. Orthodontic treatment increase value of ANB angle and, at the same time, increase of angle H. FR-III changed angle H from 5.35° to 8.25° and Y appliance from 6.60° to 7.85°, both with statistical significance p<0.001*. Patients with pseudo skeletal Class III have typical concave profile, with back position of the upper jaw. That is why upper lip is significantly posteriorly moved to the aesthetic line. FR-III approach upper lip to the aestetic line and changed distance from-5.15mm to-1.80mm. Y appliance, also, change sagittal position of the upper lip and decreased distance to the aesthetic line from-4.85mm to-3.45mm. In the whole sample lower lip was significantly back to the aesthetic line. Both appliances affect the movement of the lower lip to the aesthetic line. Y appliance changed position of the lower lip from-0.80mm to 0.30mm and FR-III changed distance of the lower lip to the aesthetic line from-1.25mm to-0.80mm. Patients with pseudo Class III have underdeveloped upper jaw and reduced height of the upper lip. Orthodontic treatment stimulated sagittal growth of the upper jaw. This allows changes in soft tissue profile and increasing the height of the upper lip. FR-III caused increasing of height of the upper lip from 21.75mm to 23.45mm, while Y appliance increased this parameter from 21.60mm to 22.30mm. Changes of position of the upper and lower lip and increasing of height of the upper lip contributes to the reduction of profile concavity [57, 58, 59]. During the period of puberty growth, changes on soft tissues are much more pronounced than on skeletal structures. Upper and lower lip and other soft tissues move down a function of time. It is important to choose the best possible treatment procedure if we want to achieve a good relationship between soft tissue and bone structures. It is important to analyse value of nasolabial angle. In patients with decreased nasolabial angle orthodontic treatment has to achieve posterior movement of the upper jaw. In cases with increased value of nasolabial angle, it is necessary to move nasomax-illary complex forward during orthodontic treatment. Orthodontic treatment caused decrease of profile concavity, increasing of height and thickness of the upper lip and anterior movement of the upper lip to the aesthetic line [60].

Patients with skeletal Class III often have infantile swalowing with anterior tongue position and oral respiration. Speech is orofacial function which last develops during individual maturation. Patients with skeletal Class III have reverse overjet. That is why articulation of interdental and labial consonants is incorrect. FR-III equally successfully corrects morphological and functional differences and contributes the correct performance of orofacial functions. FR-III significantly affects the function of swallowing and contributes to the transition from infantile to mature swallowing. In this sample (treated with FR-III) before treatment 12 patients had infantile swallowing, while 8 patients had mature swallowing. After orthodontic treatment with FR-III 13 patients had mature swallowing, while 7 had infantile swallowing. Design of FR-III prevents tongue insertion between upper and lower incisors. FR-III change activity and tongue position and it contributes changes in the function of swallowing [61]. Y appliance did not have influence on changing of swallowing function. FR-III improves articulation of interdental cionsonants, due to activity of lip muscles and changing of upper incisors inclination. Before orthodontic treatment 8 patients had correct speech and 12 patients had incorrect speech. After orthodontic treatment with FR-III 14 patients had correct speech, while 6 patients had incorrect speech. FR-III changes activity of muscles and eliminates incorrect relation between upper and lower lip.

Pancherz´s analysis explained changes on dental and skeletal structures. FR-III corrected molar relation for 3.25mm and Y appliance for 2.35mm. Relations between incisors were changed for 2.40mm when using FR-III and for 2.10mm when using Y appliance. Skeletal correction was more effective when using FR-III, for 3.30mm, while Y appliance caused skeletal correction for 1.40mm. FR-III caused skeletal correction according to stimulating of osteoblasts in periost and intensive sagittal growth of the upper jaw [62, 63, 64]. Mobile appliance caused primarily dental correction, while skeletal changes were irrelevant. Dental effects were manifested as correction of reverse overjet due to protrusion of the upper and retrusion of the lower frontal teeth.

9. Conclusion

FR-I is the most effective functional appliance in early treatment of skeletal distal bite. This appliance corrects occlusal morphology, orofacial functions and facial aesthetics. Main skeletal effects of FR-I are:

• anterior displacement and stimulation of sagittal growth of the lower jaw

• suppression of the sagittal growth of the upper jaw

• significantly increasing of length of mandibular corpus and ramus

• decreasing value of ANB angle and correction of skeletal Class II to Class I

• decreasing of vertical interjaw angle

• elimination of the pressure, application of pressure, application of pulling force and continuous activation of orofacial muscles

• increasing of sum of angles of Björk polygon and moderate backward rotation

The main dental effects of FR-I are:

• retrusion of the upper incisors

- protrusion of the lower incisors

- rotation of the occlusal plane

- mesial movement of lower posterior teeth

- distal movement of upper posterior teeth

This appliance is very comfortable for wearing, does not affect the function of speech, patients are motivated to cooperate. Treatment is very efficient, therapeutic results are stabile and tendency to relapse is minimal. That's why FR-I is the most appropriate appliance for successful early treatment of Class II divison 1 malocclusion.

Also, FR-III is one of the best choice for early orthodontic treatment of skeletal Class III caused by maxillary retrognatism. This functional appliance affects occlusal morphology, orofacial functions and facial aesthetics. In all segments FR-III is much more efficient in comparing with Y mobile appliance. Effects of this appliance are the result of stimulating of sagittal and transversal growth of the upper jaw, inhibition of growth of the lower jaw, elimination of the pressure, aplication of the pressure, tensile stress force and continuous activation of orofacial muscles. Pseudo Class III is severe skeletal problem which is transferred from the deciduous dentition to mixed and permanent dentition. If we use FR-III in early mixed dentition we avoid the use of other functional appliances during puberty growth. First therapeutic results appear after 3 to 6 months from the beginning of treatment, results are stabile, without signs of relapse, with correct protocol of wearing. The main disadvantages of this appliance are complicated preparation in dental laboratory, gracile structure, inability to repair appliance and a long duration of orthodontic therapy. The main advantages of this appliance are the possibilities of application at an early age, correction of functional and occlusal irregularities at the same time, the patient's motivation, good cooperation and comfort.

The main skeletal effects of FR-III are:

- stimulation of sagittal growth of the upper jaw

- increasing of vertical angle between upper jaw and anterior cranial base

- significant increase of length of maxilarry corpus

- inhibition of sagittal growth of the lower jaw

- increasing of vertical angle between lower jaw and anterior cranial base

- increasing value of ANB angle and correction skeletal Class III to Class I

- increasing of basal angle (B)

- increasing of sum of angles of Björk polygon and moderate backward rotation

The main dental effects of FR-III are:

- protrusion of the upper incisors

- retrusion of the lower incisors

- rotation of the occlusal plane

- distal movement of lower posterior teeth

- mesial movement of upper posterior teeth

Dental effects allow correction of reverse overjet and achieve proper overjet and correction of molar relations.

FR-III significantly alters the activity of orofacial muscles and affects the correction of swallowing and speech functions. Treatment with FR-III contributes to achieving better facial aesthetics and establishing harmony between the soft and hard tissues of the craniofacial complex.

We can recommend this functional appliance for everyday clinical practice and successful early treatment in patients with skeletal distal and mesial (pseudo Class III) bite.

Author details

Zorana Stamenković* and Vanja Raičković

*Address all correspondence to: zzokac@yahoo.com

Department of Orthodontics, Faculty of Dentisty, University of Belgrade, Serbia

References

[1] Dodić S.: Analiza morfologije i funkcije orofacijalnog kompleksa u adolescenata sa kraniomandibularnim disfunkcijama. Doktorska teza. Beograd, 2003.

[2] Battagel J.: The aetological factors in Class III malocclusion. Eur. J. Orthod. 1993; 15: 347-370.

[3] Mc Guigan D. G.: The Hapsburgs. London. WH Allen. 1966.

[4] Bishara SE. Textbook of orthodontics. W. B. Saunders; Philadelphia, 2001.

[5] O'Relly T., Yanneillo G.: Mandibular growth changes and maturation of cervical vertebrae – A longitudinal cephalometric study. Angle Orthod. 1988; 4: 179-184.

[6] Ball G, Woodside D, Tompson B, Hunter WS, Posluns J. Relationship between cervical vertebral maturation and mandibular growth. Am J Orthod Dent Orthop 2011; 139 (5): 455-461.

[7] Proffit W.B. Fields H. W., Sarver D. M.: Contemporary orthodontics. The Mosby Co. St: Louis, 2007.

[8] Almeida M. R., Henriques J. F. C., Almeida R. R., Almeida-Pedrin R. R., Ursi W.: Treatment effects produced by the Bionator appliance. Comparison with an untreated Class II sample. Eur. J. Orthod. 2004; 26: 65-72.

[9] Carlos Flores-Mir and Paul W. Major: A systematic review of cephalometric facial soft tissue changes with the Activator and Bionator appliances in Class II division 1 subjects. Eur. J. Orthod. 2006; 28: 586-593.

[10] Faltin K. J., Faltin R. M., Baccetti T., Franchi L., Ghiozzi B., McNamara J. A. Jr.: Long-term effectiveness and treatment timing for Bionator therapy. Angle Orthod. 2003; 73 (3): 221-230.

[11] Hotz R.: Orthodontics in daily practice. Bern, Switzerland, Huber. 1974.

[12] Isaacson K. G., Muir J. D., Reed R. T. Removable orthodontic Appliances, Oxford, 2002.

[13] Fränkel R., Fränkel Ch.: Orofacial Orthopaedics with the Function Regulator. Karger, Basel – Munchen –Paris – London – New York – New Delhi – Singapore – Tokyo – Sydney, 1989.

[14] Fränkel R.: Funktionskieferorthopadie und der Mundvorhof als Papparatus Basis, VEB Verl., Berlin, 1967.

[15] Fränkel R.: A functional approach to orofacial orthopaedics. Br. J. Orthod. 1980; 7: 41-51

[16] Kanas R. J., Carapezza L., Kanas S. J.: Treatment Clasification of Class III Malocclusion. The Journal of Clinical Pediatric Dentistry. 2008; 33(2): 175-186.

[17] Baik H. S., Jee S. H., Lee K. J., Oh T. K.: Treatment effect of Frankel functional regulator III in children with class III malocclusions. Am. J. Orthod. Dentofacial Orthop. 2004; 125: 294-301.

[18] Stamenković Z.: Klinički efekti primene Fränkel-ovih regulatora funkcije u terapiji distalnog i mezijalnog zagrižaja. Doktorska disertacija. Beograd, 2011.

[19] Almeida M. R., Henriques J. F. C. and Ursi W.: Comparative study of the Frankel (FR-2) and bionator appliances in the treatment of Class II malocclusion. Am. J. Orthod. Dentofacial Orthop. 2002; 121: 458-466.

[20] Araujo A. M., Buschang P. H., Melo A. C. M.: Adaptive condylar growth and mandibular remodeling changes with bionator therapy – an implant study. Eur. J. Orthod. 2004; 26: 515-522.

[21] Chen J. Y., Will L., Neiderman R.: Analysis of efficacy of functional appliances on mandibular growth. Am. J. Orthod. Dentofacial orthop. 2002; 122: 470-476.

[22] Yamin-Lacouture C., Woodside D.G., Sectakof P.A., Sessle B.J.: The action of three types of functional appliances on the activity of the masticatory muscles. Am. J. Orthod. Dentofacial Orthop. 1997; 112: 560-572.

[23] Martins R. P., Martin J. C., Martins L. P., Buschang P. H.: Skeletal and dental components of Class II correction with the bionator and removable headgear splint appliances. Am. J. Orthod. Dentofacial Orthop. 2008; 134: 732-741.

[24] Chadwick S.M., Aird C., Taylor S., Bearn D.R.: Functional regulator treatment of Class II division 1 malocclusions. Eur. J. Orthod. 2001; 23: 495-505.

[25] Barton S., Cook P. A.: Predicting functional appliance treatment outcome in Class II malocclusions – a rewiew. Am. J. Orthod. Dentofacial Orthop. 1997; 112: 282-286.

[26] Cevidanes L. et al: Clinical outcomes of Fränkel appliance therapy assessed with a counterpart analysis. Am. J. orthod. Dentofacial Orthop. 2003; 123: 379-387.

[27] Moreira Melo A. C., dos Santos-Pinto A., da Rosa Martins J. C., Martins L. P., Sakima M. T.: Orthopedic and orthodontic components of Class II, division 1 malocclusion correction with Balters Bionator: A cephalometric study with metallic implants. World J. Orthod. 2003; 4: 273-242.

[28] Rodrigues de Almeida M., Castanha Henriques J. F., Rodrigues de Almeida R., Ursi W.: Treatment effects produced bz Fränkel appliance in patients with Class II, division 1 malocclusion. Angle Orthod. 2002; 72 (5): 418-425.

[29] Falck F., Fränkel R.: Clinical relevance of step-by-step mandibular advancement in the treatment of mandibular retrusion using the Fränkel appliance. Am. J. Orthod. Dentofacial Orthop. 1989; 96: 333-341.

[30] Thieme KM, Nägerl H, Hahn W, Ihlow D, Kubein D. Variations in cyclic mandibular movements during treatment of Class II malocclusions with removable functional appliances. Eur J Orthod 2011: 33(6): 628-635.

[31] Patel H. P., Moseley H. C., Noar J. H.: Cephalometric determinants of successful functional appliance therapy. Angle Orthod. 2002; 72: 410-417.

[32] Battagel J. M.: Profile changes in Class II, division 1 malocclusions: a comparison of the effects of Edgewise and Fränkel appliance therapy. Eur. J. Orthod. 1989; 11: 243-253.

[33] Battagel J. M.: The relationship between hard and soft tissue changes following treatment og Class II division 1 malocclusions using Edgewise and Fränkel appliance techniques, Eur. J. Orthod. 1990; 12: 154-165.

[34] [34]Quintao C., Helena I., Brunharo V. P., Menezes R. C., Almeida M. A. O: Soft tissue facial profile changes following functional appliance therapy. Eur. J. Orthod. 2006; 28: 35-41.

[35] Creekmore T. D., Radney L.J.: Frankel appliance therapy: orthopedic or orthodontic? Am. J. Orthod. 1983; 83:89-108.

[36] Janson G.R.P., Alegria Toruno J.L., Rodrigez Martins D., Henriques J.F.C., de Freitas M.R.: Class II treatment effects of the Fränkel appliance. Eur. J. Orthod. 2003; 25: 301-309.

[37] Read M. J. F.: The integration of functional and fixed appliance treatment. Am. J. Orthod. 2001; 28 (1): 13-18.

[38] Woodside D. G.: Do functional appliances have an orthopedic effect? Am. J. Orthod. Dentofacial Orthop. 1998; 113:11.

[39] Pancherz H., Zieber K., Hoyer B.: Cephalometric characteristics of Class II division 1 and Class II division 2 malocclusions: a comparative study in children, Angle Orthod. 1997; 67: 111-120.

[40] Rushforth C. D., Gordon P. H., Aird J. C.: Skeletal and dental changes following the use of the Frankel funkcional regulator. Br. J. Orthod. 1999; 26:127-134.

[41] Bacetti T. et al.: Skeletal effects of early treatment of Class III malocclusion. Am. J. Orthod. Dentofac. Orthop. 1998; 113: 333 – 343.

[42] Levin A. S., McNamara J. A. Jr., Franchi L., Baccetti T., Frankel C.: Short-term and long-term treatment outcomes with the FR-3 appliance of Frankel. Am. J. Orthod. Dentofacial Orthop. 2008; 134: 513-524.

[43] Miethke R. R., Lindenau S., Dietrich K.: The effect of Fränkel's function regulator type III on the apical base. Eur. J. Orthod.2003; 25: 311-318.

[44] Negi A., Singla A., Mahajan V.: Effects of Maxilarry Protraction And Frankel Appliance Therapy On Craniofacial Structures And Pharyngeal Airway. Indian Journal of Dental Sciences. 2013; 5(5): 30-33.

[45] Pangrazio-Kulbersh V., Berger J., Kersten G.: Effects of protraction mechanics on the midface. Am. J. Orthod. Dentofacial Orthop. 1998; 114: 484-491.

[46] Seehra J., Fleming P. S., Mandall N., DiBiase A. T.: A comparison of two different techniques for early correction of Class III malocclusion. The Angle Orthodontist. 2012; 82(1): 96-101.

[47] Fränkel R: Maxillary retrusion in Class III and treatment with the functional corrector III. Trans. Eur. Orthod. Soc. 1970; 46: 249-259.

[48] Almeida M. R., Almeida R. R., Oltramari-Navarro P. V., Conti A. C., Navarro R de L, Camacho J. G.: Early treatment of Class III malocclusion: 10-year clinical follow-up. J Appl Oral Sci.: 2011; 19: 431-439.

[49] Zentner A., Doll G. M., Peylo S. M.: Morphological parameters as predictors of successful correction of Class III malocclusion. Eur. J. Orthod. 2001; 23: 383-392.

[50] Santos-Pinto A. D., Paulin R. F., Moreira Melo A. C.: Pseudo-Class III treatment with reverse traction: case report. Journal of Clinical Pediatric Dentistry. 2001; 25 (4): 264-274.

[51] Ulgen M., Firatli S.: The effects of Fränkel's function regulator on the Class III malocclusions. Am. J. Orthod. 1994; 105: 561-567.

[52] Oltramari-Navarro P. V. P., Almeida R. R., Conti A. C., Navaro R de L. et al: Early treatment Protocol for Skeletal Class III Malocclusion. Brazilian Dental Journal. 2013; 24(2): 167-173.

[53] Toffol L. D., Pavoni C., Bacceti T., Franchi L. and Cozza P.: Orthopedic treatment outcomes in Class III malocclusion. The Angle Orthod. 2008; 78: 561-573.

[54] Giancotti A., Maselli A., Mampieri G. and Spano E.: Pseudo-Class III malocclusion treatment with Balters´ bionator. Br. Orthodontic Soc. 2003; 30 (3): 203-215.

[55] Loh M. K., Kerr W. J. S.: The function regulator III: effects and indications for use. Br. J. Orthod. 1985; 12: 153-157.

[56] Kapur A., Chawla H. S., Utreja A., Goyla A.: Early Class III occlusal tendency in children and its selective management, Journal of the Indian Society of Pedodontics and Preventive Dentistry. 2008; 26 (3): 107-113.

[57] Stamenković Z., Nedeljković N.: Karakteristike mekotkivnog profila kod pacijenata sa III skeletnom klasom. Stomatološki glasnik Srbije, 2006. Vol. 53, 166-173.

[58] Zhao G., Sha L., Chang B.: Soft tissue profile changes by Frankel-III appliance on correcting Angle Class III malocclusion in mixed dentition. Shanghai Journal of Stomatology. 2011; 20(2): 201-203.

[59] Kerr W. J., Ten Have T. R.: Changes in soft tissue profile during the treatment of Class III malocclusion. Br. J. Orthod. 1987; 14(4): 243-249.

[60] Prashanth C. S., Dinesh M. R., Akshai Shetty K. R.: Class III – Three way approach, a review of contemporary treatment modalities. Journal of International Oral Health. 2010; 2(1): 27-30.

[61] Robertson N. R. E.: An examination of treatment changes in children treated with the function regulator of Frankel. Am. J. Orthod. 1983; 83: 299-310.

[62] Chen F., Terada K., Wu L., Saito I.: Longitudinal evaluation of the intermaxilarry relationship in Class III malocclusions. Angle Orthod. 2006; 76: 955-961.

[63] Standt C. B., Kiliaridis S.: Different skeletal types underlying Class III malocclusion in a random population. Am J Orthod Dentofacial Orthop. 2009; 136: 715-721.

[64] Zentner A., Doll G. M.: Size discrepancy of apical bases and treatment success in Angle Class III malocclusion. Journal of Orofacial Orthopedics 2001; 62: 97-106.

9

Periodontal Disease — A Physician's Viewpoint

Myers J.B.

1. Introduction

From the physician's viewpoint teeth and the periodontal framework are relatively ignored. How many physicians actually inspect the teeth of their patients let alone their patients' gums? Increasingly though, awareness of integration and holistic appreciation of organ function has penetrated the formal divides that separate clinical practice according to body parts and organ function.

2. A deeper look in a clinical context

Metabolic function that is general and common to all body parts, and the inflammatory basis of disease highlight the commonality that underlies these processes. It is therefore not surprising to find that, in theory, changes in nail capillaries reflect capillary integrity in other body parts and signs of inflammatory disease that is present elsewhere may be seen in peripheral nail capillaries.

It has been proposed that periodontal disease is a factor resulting in inflammatory changes, raised C-reactive protein levels and loss of capillaries through inflammatory thrombotic events that results in increased cardiovascular risk and cognitive loss [1], as all body parts including brain become affected [2]. Thus if an association exists between capillary loss and rarefaction with cognitive decline and silent or ischaemic cardiomyopathy and ischaemic heart disease periodontal disease is a risk factor that needs to be considered. Similarly stroke occurs more commonly after an infection such as upper respiratory infection or urinary tract infection [3]. Thus inflammation resulting in stroke may also arise as a result of periodontal disease [1].

Microcirculatory changes involving capillary may be attributable to periodontal disease on the basis of inflammatory products being generated on a persistent basis [1,2]. There is also the theoretical proposition that large vessels too are or become affected. Atheroma formation may be an inflammatory process [4]. It could result from the interaction of inflammatory proteins or monocytes acting on a dysfunctional endothelial surface such as may affect the lining of major blood vessels in the presence of underlying atheromatous change. These inflammatory cytokines [interleukin [IL]-1, IL-6] may be generated by periodontal disease and be linked to atheroma formation [5].

The effect on both micro-circulation i.e. capillaries and on the large vessels could result in increasing blood pressure and aggravate hypertension or even cause it if damage sufficient to impair capillary reserve capacity occurs, on challenge with a higher sodium intake, leads to the development of hypertension [6,7]. Similarly, renal effects would lead to renal impairment and even failure, as occurs in autoimmune [8] or hypertensive disease [9,10] or result in stroke and cerebral infarction or white matter degenerative change that manifest as vascular dementia [11] and even states of confusion depending on the severity and acuteness of the microcirculatory rarefaction and /or dysfunction.

Thus periodontal disease affects microcirculation integrity as well as larger vessels predisposing to cardiovascular risk through microvascular rarefaction and atheroma formation. Microvascular changes are themselves the cause of large vessel changes. Dysfunction or loss of perivascular capillaries affect large vessel compliance [12] in much the same way that periodontal vessels have an effect on dental health and function.

3. Treatment — Preventive, prophylactic and after the fact

Treatment of risk factors and complications such as stroke or cognitive loss must address the question is periodontal disease present. Diabetic disease is also related to this.

4. Periodontal health and general health and wellbeing

Periodontal disease causes halitosis and dentition. The presentation of a person relies on the ability to smile and is enhanced by having a set of healthy teeth and healthy breath. In Jewish law, bad breadth is a sufficient reason for divorce. A smile is everything. It secures a job, makes friends, is high profile as well as high society and it ensures the willingness of others to help when behaviour is amicable and is accompanied by a smile, that, I contend, is as important a factor as incontinence or continence in either resulting in institutionalised care or willing helpers to assist in home based care if that is their preferred choice rather than institutionalisation.

Mouth breathing: upper respiratory complaints are the source. Chronic upper respiratory blockage leads to snoring and poor sleep. It causes those who cannot breathe through their nose to gulp, not chew their food and to put on weight. The answer is to clear the nose with steam inhalation and to practice "how to breathe when you eat", Breathe in then out then insert a small amount of food into your mouth and chew, then swallow before you breathe in again, through your nose. Eat with your mouth closed and practice breathing in through your nose using the abdominal transverse muscles and diaphragm to aerate the lungs through your nose. It is not uncommon for these people to present with what appears to be an asthma attack on a cold night. The dentist, too, as well as the physician, has to be aware of this [13].

What does dental form tell you? By this I mean the effect of thumb sucking, which is a transient phase, but could persist or recur, indicates a psychological effect or emotional disturbance that could influence adult behaviour, which is notional on my part, not researched. Yet, when the individual takes steps to overcome this, to have the cosmetic treatments that correct this, they are at the same time overcoming the insecurity that led to the "buck-teeth" and building confidence to deal with situations from within. This is healthy and surely indicates the place of cosmetic dentistry in the recovery motivated by inner strength to change, i.e. the place of dental treatments in psychological and emotional wellbeing. For the same reason, treatments that overcome or help to contain periodontal disease that cause bad breath through simple oral hygiene, especially in those patients predisposed to this, whether through mouth breathing or on anti-epileptic agents that produce gum hypertrophy, such as phenytoin, is important.

Smoking habit and oral health. I believe that is not uncommon that people who mouth breathe smoke. In this situation smoking warms the air and damages the cilia on the bronchial cell lining. The reflex that responds to cold air with a cough is therefore overcome and mucus production in the bronchi remains there as the cilia of ciliated bronchial cells that are paralysed cannot move it up. Smoking also discolours the teeth, pipe smoking breaks them. When the sinuses are blocked the air cannot be warmed nor humidified. Treatment may be given for asthmatic attack or long term for asthma, that may be an incorrect assessment of events. Steroid inhalator therapy may result in fungal overgrowth in the oral mucosa without therapeutic benefit either long term or during an acute attack [13].

Too many sweets. But its not the fruit. Its the sticky stuff and sticky stuff combined with acids that corrode or vehicles such as flour that stick to one's teeth.

Geriatric dentistry: care of the elderly includes attention to oral health and diet. Access to clinic and to the dental chair have to be user friendly. Assistance may be needed. Lowering the dental chair to a convenient level to get onto and off, safely. Head up tilt and back support may be required. Rheumatoid arthritis does affect the neck, so neck extension is to be prevented.

Visits to nursing homes and now routine; medications and poly-pharmacy remain sources of notable concern. All medications cannot be listed here. The newer oral anticoagulants [NOAC's] used as prophylaxis against stroke in patients with non-valvular atrial fibrillation, e.g. Dabigatran, a direct thrombin inhibitor [DTI] and Apixaban, Rivaroxaban [Factor Xa inhibitors] are increasingly being used to replace Warfarin/Vitamin K depleting anticoagulants [14]. Since new information is becoming available at a rapid pace, an "EHRA" web site with the latest updated information accompanies the guide able to be accessed on its website [www.NOACforAF.eu]. It also contains links to the ESC AF Guidelines, a key message pocket booklet, print-ready files for a proposed universal NOAC anticoagulation card, and feedback possibilities. Side-effect hazards include anti-fungal agents and calcium channel blockers, Verapamil and Diltiazem, which increases the level and effects of NOAC's manifold as do "ketokonazole" and like anti-fungal medications that render unacceptable NOAC's risk of haemorrhage. Quinine also increases the level of drug and risk. Partial thromboplastin time may be used to check Dabigatran effects. Renal function also affects the dose and needs to be regularly checked [up to six monthly]. Refer to www.NOACforAF.eu]. Ceasing treatment for dental treatments for at least twelve hours is advised, see paragraph 10 of the guide.

It is important to hand to the elderly patient written instructions for the patient if they are able and/or to a carer or accompanying person who may also be able to supervise, assist if necessary and give to you information regarding what other medications the person is taking, to bring in the dosette box, which is pre-packed by the pharmacy or by the carer or by the patient who is able and willing – it's a good mental exercise, as well as non-medications or unprescribed treatments.

Nutritional intake and health; role of carer; dental replacements – inserts, implants for nutrition and comfort; the importance of nutrition and type of foods available as well as types of diet, vitamised, soft can maintain health and prevent ill-health.

Aging is the inexorable loss of functional reserve capacity. There is a functional metabolic reserve, that could apply to anaesthetic agents, number of teeth, ability to chew, ability to swallow and ability to transfer to a chair, which maintains independence as the person is able to get onto and off a toilet and to mobilise. Exercise and nutrition are central to maintaining independence.

Cosmetic dentistry in the elderly is now available but not the only reason to undertake having new implants. At ninety three years, my mother chose to have implants as her dentures bothered her so much. Painful dentures can ruin any person's life, spoil one's appreciation of food, cause ulcers as everyone knows but also determine what one can eat or not eat. Loss of weight through poor dentition or ill fitting dentures can have devastating results, leading to a fall by having a mat in the wrong place and not lifting up one's feet, just once. Fracture, having to recuperate and being placed is the greatest risk of being admitted to a hospital, at least in Australia, where the maxim, we have a duty of care – to maintain safety" overtakes the right of privilege and free choice. Here, the word of an expert, whom the patient only trusts, is shunned by those with agenda's of their own, including seeking power and feeling of self importance. With less knowledge and greater inferiority everyone has their say. The Office of the Public Advocate, the bureaucrats on Tribunals and Medical Boards, who know less and are lesser individuals because they wish to control those who have made it, live it and enjoy it. What has this got to do with oral health? The answer is nutrition, trust, and confidence and an ability to communicate positively to one's environment, which is more likely to happen when one has a smile and a good set of teeth and friends in support. It will determine who will be prepared to care for you and who will not. It will ensure that where you live is where you wish to live and with whom.

Inflammation and infection is not as obvious in the elderly as immune mechanisms are not as intense, or able to marshalled, but tissue turgor is also not as dense and therefore pain is less. On the other hand recovery takes time. Even after extractions one needs to be cared for. One ought to take in higher protein drinks before and to continue to do so afterwards. The advent of bisphosphonates, which inhibit osteoclast recruitment and reduces bone loss in the treatment of osteoporosis and secondary prevention in cases with fracture of the femur or vertebrae has resulted in fear of osteonecrosis of the jaw [15], which is more likely to occur in patients who are receiving chemotherapy. Pretreatment dental surgery is suggested as well as use of antibiotics and an oral antiseptic solution when the condition occurs to treat and control pain [15].

5. Social dentistry

I have likened the loss of a tooth to the social situation of an elderly person. When one loses a friend one also loses support and one's own position becomes more vulnerable. This leads to lack of confidence, to isolation from society and to becoming depressed. Living in a residential home is akin to having a set of dentures. They are not yours, but they are there and do provide some comfort, but not always.

Tooth extraction is a metaphor for diminution of social interaction; support and social functioning in the elderly; isolation and depression, effect of loss and deprivation, while restoration is akin to the effect of nutrition on wellbeing, psychological, physical and spiritual.

Behaviour and institutionalisation: The effect of oral health, hygiene and behaviour can ensure that you will stay longer in your own home and even die there in familiar memory clad surroundings. Nothing insures this better than behaviour characterised by appreciation, thanks and a smile.

In old age, in adults and teens; the effect is the same. Confidence, radiating happiness and achievement are related to dental pride and appearance.

6. Oral function as a driver in social evolution

Stomal drive in evolution. Food and water intake determines survival.

Setting down roots led to stomatal development; to vegetative and sessile development.

Stomal development led to cortical development and permitted mobility.

Senses in animals included two eyes and two ears. Dentition permitted there to be one mouth for fluids and solids and determined strength development on the basis of what could be eaten when caught, the consistency of foods. Eyes and ears were used as warning signs to prevent being eaten and to survey what could be eaten or caught.

Amphibian and reptilian evolutionary dichotomy occurred as amphibians developed a buccal respiration pattern, using the floor of the mouth to create air movement into and out of the lungs, whereas reptiles developed ribs and birds developed air sacks in those ribs to lighten the weight and developed beaks as the driver rather than alligator teeth, though the Cretaceous creatures, Pterosaurs, that flew such as Pterodactylus had a small number of teeth, while Pteranodon was completely toothless. This fact, combined with Pteranodon's vaguely albatross-like build, has led paleontologists to conclude that this pterosaur flew along the seashores of late Cretaceous North America and fed mostly on fish [16].

Snakes developed the tooth to the utmost by having a venom ejaculation mechanism in them used in forward fanged snakes such as Viperidae [vipers] to blind or poison their prey before they ate them. Ear ossicles later incorporated into the middle ear in higher vertebrates, that are part of the mandibular system in snakes enabled the snake to dislocate his mandible to swallow large prey whole, and their fangs to catch prey, as least in the forward fanged snakes, whose body lengths are shorter than constrictors, rather than masticate. The extra ossicles also permitted vibration detection in preparedness to catch their prey as well as to swallow it, indicating the economy of form in relation to function that appears to be a formula for successful evolution; the combining of survival mechanisms: energy acquisition, through ingestion and metabolism, which also requires excretion, to live, grow and mate and energy expenditure to escape or, alternatively to develop further and adapt.

In the invertebrate world helminths developed suckers and they became tapeworm parasites, while special insertion of sperm techniques used by spiders ended by self sacrifice, with the male being eaten to provide ready nourishment for the newly fertilised eggs, taking the survival pitch of stomal drive to its ultimate.

Years ago, the rabbis recognised that food which is visually tempting increases appetite [17]. Plants use colour to attract insects to feast on the nectar as the lure to pollinate inadvertently and by the design of the plant while the insects eat. The latter example has a message – when you help others eat by providing nectar and food, they share in the benefits that you reproduce, which ensures that their progeny have energy in the form of nectar to eat.

Primal instinct and stomal drive – in the 21st century. A primal instinct demands our focus. In today's world while success can be founded on dental presentation, it can also be one's undoing, when stomal drive is for one's own sake, rather than for survival.

Obsession with desire that may attend one who has achieved success, in detracting from the focus of what one eats and gratitude for every morsel that appreciation of survival demands, results in a change in priorities, such that desire overtakes survival. Dependency results, as does pleasure drive and desire, to hedonism, loss of survival focus and breakdown.

It is true that eating can be fashioned to ensure body health and looks. It can also induce anorexia or bulimia. We need to be in tune with our primal instincts. They are a survival mechanism. Stomal health, includes oral hygiene and cortical awareness.

The stomal society. Society has cultural values that are tied to eating patterns. Nations are distinguished by their cultural or national cuisine. Japanese food is unique to Japan. Middle

Eastern food is particular to the middle east. African food to Africa. It ties us to the land. Chinese food is unique to Chinese. Is it fair to ask whether Italian culture would be what it is today if Marco Polo (1254-1324) had not brought back noodles from the Far East?

Cultures with traditions that incorporate food as symbols of significance and ethical values, as is the case with traditional Jewish customs, ensures that there is focus on survival as they are enjoyed and partaken to ensure history and moral values and ethics of daily life are transmitted to future generations. Therefore they do survive and can impart ethical values and morality to the world, for generations.

Stomal drive remains the focus during development as well as into old age. The application of implant techniques to old age in order to be able to masticate and enjoy a wholesome meal will ensure longer life and a more pleasing one. On the other hand cosmetic dentistry which forsakes nutritional and masticatory functions may shorten lifespan by changing focus and permitting distraction from survival to creep in.

7. Lips and buccal function

Although the lips have not been addressed in this chapter, lip function and the cheeks, ensures swallowing without spillage, as occurs in lower motor neurone facial palsy or paralysis. Lips have a prehensile function working with the tongue in almost mitten like clasp that enables giraffe to selectively eat the leaves they desire from the top of trees. Lips also reveal features of human emotion and desire. They also permit breath-holding and labial sounds.

8. General systems theory and stomal drive

The concept of the "constancy of the milieu extérieur"[7] i.e. maintaining one's environment in terms of Eco-social© harmony [18] even in response to change, this means ensuring diversity of activity, and diversity of flora and fauna. External milieu is also the lymph and plasma bathing cells [7]. What ensures this? Oral hygiene, oral health and what passes through it, liquids, solids, sounds and words.

9. Conclusion

Oral health and development determine both quality of life and quantity, as a survival mechanism essential for life the importance of stomal function for physical and emotional wellbeing as well as social functioning has been understated in the past. In addition stomal drive as a evolutionary mechanism has not been appreciated or previously understood in terms of both plant (stomata) and of invertebrate and vertebrate, animal, evolution and development, on land, in fresh water and the sea.

Author details

Myers J.B.*

Address all correspondence to: rebdoc1@bigpond.net.au

Department of Medical Science, Wellspring's Universal Environment P/L, Australia

References

[1] Myers JB. Infection, periodontal disease, inflammation, vascular (capillary) injury and cognitive decline with ageing: an hypothesis. J Neurological Sciences. 2005, 236 (Suppl.1) p518, P1650.

[2] Myers JB. "Capillary Band Width", "the Nail Sign: A clinical Marker of inflammation, vascular integrity, cognition and age. Personal Viewpoint and Hypothesis. Journal of the Neurological Sciences, Official Bulletin of the World Federation of Neurology, Suppl. 2009, 283(1-2) pp.86-90 Elsevier Publications, NY.

[3] Smeeth L, Thomas SL, Hall AJ, Hubbard R, Farrington P, Vallance P. Risk of Myocardial Infarction and Stroke after Acute Infection or Vaccination. N Engl J Med 2004;351:2611-8.

[4] Hansson GK. Immune Mechanisms in Atherosclerosis. Arteriosclerosis, thrombosis and Vascular Biology. 2001; 21: 1876-1890 doi: 10.1161/hq1201.100220

[5] Beck J, Garcia R, Heiss G, Vokonas PS, Offenbacher S. Periodontal Disease and Cardiovascular Disease. Journal of Periodontology 1996; 67(10s):1123-1137. doi:10.1902/jop.1996.67.10s.1123

[6] Myers, JB. "Sodium Sensitivity" in Man. Medical Hypotheses. 1987; 23: 265-276.

[7] Myers, JB. Biochemical response to change in the environment and the nature of "essential" hypertension. Medical Hypotheses. 1982; 9: 241-257.

[8] Kronbichler A, Mayer G. Renal involvement in autoimmune connective tissue diseases. BMC Medicine. http://www.biomedcentral.com/1741-7015/11/95

[9] Ebringer A, Doyle AE. Raised Serum IgG Levels in Hypertension. Brit Med J. 1970;2:146-148.

[10] Daniel W. Trott and David G. Harrison The immune system in hypertension. doi: 10. 1152/advan.00063.2013 Adv Physiol Educ March 1, 2014 vol. 38 no. 1 20-24.

[11] Myers JB. Sodium intake, cognitive decline and Ageing. Sixth international Congress on Vascular Dementia, Barcelona Spain. 2009; November 19-22. Abstract p83. www.Kenes.com/vascular.

[12] Stefanidis C, Vlachopoulos C, Karayannacos P, Boudoulas H, Stratos C, Filippides T, Agapitos M, Toutouzas P. Effect of Vasa Vasorum Flow on structure and Function of the Aorta in Experimental Animals. Circulation 1995; 91; 2669-2678.

[13] Myers JB. COPD exacerbations. What else is wrong with the patient? An internist's viewpoint for the benefit of patients. Internal Medicine Society of Australia and New Zealand (IMSANZ) 2011 Annual Scientific Meeting. Lorne, Vic, Australia. November 11-13, 2011.

[14] Heidbuchel H, Verhamme P, Alings M, Antz M, Hacke W, Oldgren J, Sinnaeve P, Camm AJ, Kirchhof P. EHRA Practical Guide on the use of new oral anticoagulants in patients with non-valvular atrial fibrillation: executive summary. European Heart Journal doi:10.1093/eurheartj/eht134

[15] Marx RE, Sawatari Y, Fortin M, Broumand V. Bisphosphonate-Induced Exposed Bone [Osteonecrosis/Osteopetrosis] of the Jaws: Risk Factors, Recognition, Prevention, and Treatment. J Oral Maxillofac Surg 2005; 63:1567–1575.

[16] Strauss B. 10 Facts About Pterodactyls. Everything You Need to Know About Pterodactylus and Pteranodon. http://dinosaurs.about.com/od/dinosaurbasics/a/pterodactyl-facts.htm (accessed 16 September 2014)

[17] Yoma, 74-5. In: Ayin Yaacov.

[18] Myers JB. The Eco-society or Eco-social© environment and heart disease. A General Systems Approach. PM358. World Heart Federation's World Congress of Cardiology 2014. May 4-7, Melbourne, Australia.

Permissions

All chapters in this book were first published in ETOHSD, by InTech Open; hereby published with permission under the Creative Commons Attribution License or equivalent. Every chapter published in this book has been scrutinized by our experts. Their significance has been extensively debated. The topics covered herein carry significant findings which will fuel the growth of the discipline. They may even be implemented as practical applications or may be referred to as a beginning point for another development.

The contributors of this book come from diverse backgrounds, making this book a truly international effort. This book will bring forth new frontiers with its revolutionizing research information and detailed analysis of the nascent developments around the world.

We would like to thank all the contributing authors for lending their expertise to make the book truly unique. They have played a crucial role in the development of this book. Without their invaluable contributions this book wouldn't have been possible. They have made vital efforts to compile up to date information on the varied aspects of this subject to make this book a valuable addition to the collection of many professionals and students.

This book was conceptualized with the vision of imparting up-to-date information and advanced data in this field. To ensure the same, a matchless editorial board was set up. Every individual on the board went through rigorous rounds of assessment to prove their worth. After which they invested a large part of their time researching and compiling the most relevant data for our readers.

The editorial board has been involved in producing this book since its inception. They have spent rigorous hours researching and exploring the diverse topics which have resulted in the successful publishing of this book. They have passed on their knowledge of decades through this book. To expedite this challenging task, the publisher supported the team at every step. A small team of assistant editors was also appointed to further simplify the editing procedure and attain best results for the readers.

Apart from the editorial board, the designing team has also invested a significant amount of their time in understanding the subject and creating the most relevant covers. They scrutinized every image to scout for the most suitable representation of the subject and create an appropriate cover for the book.

The publishing team has been an ardent support to the editorial, designing and production team. Their endless efforts to recruit the best for this project, has resulted in the accomplishment of this book. They are a veteran in the field of academics and their pool of knowledge is as vast as their experience in printing. Their expertise and guidance has proved useful at every step. Their uncompromising quality standards have made this book an exceptional effort. Their encouragement from time to time has been an inspiration for everyone.

The publisher and the editorial board hope that this book will prove to be a valuable piece of knowledge for researchers, students, practitioners and scholars across the globe.

List of Contributors

Ana Isabel García-Kass, Juan Antonio García-Núñez and Victoriano Serrano-Cuenca
Department of Stomatology III, School of Dentistry, Complutense University of Madrid, Madrid, Spain

Petra Surlin
University of Medicine and Pharmacy of Craiova, Faculty of Dental Medicine, Department of Periodontology, Romania

Anne Marie Rauten
University of Medicine and Pharmacy of Craiova, Faculty of Dental Medicine, Department of Orthodontics, Romania

Mihai Raul Popescu
University of Medicine and Pharmacy of Craiova, Faculty of Dental Medicine, Department of Occlusal Sciences, Romania

Constantin Daguci
University of Medicine and Pharmacy of Craiova, Faculty of Dental Medicine, Department of Oral Health, Romania

Maria Bogdan
University of Medicine and Pharmacy of Craiova, Faculty of Pharmacy, Department of Pharmacology, Romania

Mourad Sebbar and Zouhair Abidine
Hospital Moulay Abdellah, Mohammedia, Morocco

Narjisse Laslami and Zakaria Bentahar
Department of orthodontics, Faculty of dentistry, Casablanca, Morocco

Belma Işık Aslan and Neslihan Üçüncü
Gazi University, Faculty of Dentistry, Department of Orthodontics, Ankara, Turkey

Ileana Monica Baniță and Cristina Munteanu
Department of Dentistry, University of Medicine and Pharmacy, Craiova, Romania

Anca Berbecaru-Iovan, Camelia Elena Stănciulescu, Ana Marina Andrei and Cătălina Gabriela Pisoschi
Department of Pharmacy, University of Medicine and Pharmacy, Craiova, Romania

Hakima Aghoutan, Sana Alami, Farid El Quars and Farid Bourzgui
Department of Dento-facial Orthopedic, Faculty of Dental Medicine, Hassan II University of Casablanca, Morocco

Samir Diouny
Chouaib Doukkali University, Faculty of Letters & Human Sciences, El Jadida, Morocco

Andréa Cristina Barbosa da Silva, Diego Romário da Silva, Sabrina Avelar de Macedo Ferreira and Sandra Aparecida Marinho
Graduate Program in Dentistry, Center of Sciences, Technology and Health, State University of Paraiba, UEPB, Araruna, Paraíba, Brazil

Andeliana David de Sousa Rodrigues
Graduate Program in Dentistry, Integrated College of Patos, FIP, Patos, Paraíba, Brazil

Allan de Jesus Reis Albuquerque
Brazilian Northeast Network on Biotechnology, RENORBIO, Federal University of Paraiba, UFPB, João Pessoa, Paraíba, Brazil

Zorana Stamenković and Vanja Raičković
Department of Orthodontics, Faculty of Dentisty, University of Belgrade, Serbia

Myers J.B.
Department of Medical Science, Wellspring's Universal Environment P/L, Australia

Index

www.ingramcontent.com/pod-product-compliance
Lightning Source LLC
Chambersburg PA
CBHW062001190326
41458CB00009B/2938